I Am Interrupting This Program...

I Am Interrupting This Program

...and other writings by

Mary Goulding, M.S.W.

Zeig, Tucker & Theisen, Inc.
Phoenix Arizona

Library of Congress Cataloging-in-Publication Data
Goulding, Mary.

I am interrupting this program ...and other writings by Mary Goulding, M.S.W.

p. cm.
ISBN 978-1-934442-21-0

1. Psychotherapy 2. Transactional Analysis I. Title

Published by

ZEIG, TUCKER & THEISEN, INC.
3618 North 24th Street
Phoenix, AZ 85016

Manufactured in the United States of America

Acknowledgements

My thanks to:

Marti B Kranzberg, PhD, and Moon Kerson, PhD, editors of the *Journal of Transactional Analysis* (1998 - 2002). Some of the articles in this book began as Journal articles.

Inger Acking for her computer expertise, enthusiasm, and good suggestions.

All members of the International Transactional Analysis Association, the United States of America Transactional Analysis Association, and the Redecision Therapy Association for keeping our therapy alive.

Thanks forever to Bob Goulding, who was my mentor, therapy partner, husband and love.

Contents

ONE

Transactional Analysis and Redecision Therapy*

*The editors of *Redecision Therapy* journal asked me to explain what aspects of redecision therapy and practice are derived from transactional analysis. This chapter is taken from the article I wrote in response.

Transactional Analysis Theory

Eric Berne, founder of transactional analysis, with the assistance of members of the San Francisco Social Psychiatry Seminars (1962-1970), put together the structure of transactional analysis: ego states, transactions, games, injunctions, decisions, scripts, and strokes.

Ego states: Parent, Adult, and Child. This aspect of transactional analysis is now known worldwide. Statements such as, "Use your Adult" (almost always a Parental request), "That's my Parent talking," "My Child needs love (or a classier hotel room)," are commonly said by lay people who may never have heard of Eric Berne. Support groups are based on the victimized "inner child." If we should set ourselves the task of discovering all mention of parent, adult, and child ego states in scientific and popular literature today, I think we would be amazed to discover how widely the concept of ego states has spread.

Berne wrote of structural ego states: parents' parent, adult, and child in the Parent; the Adult; the archaic parent, adult (little professor), and primitive child in the Child. He also described functional ego states: nurturing and critical (prejudiced) Parent, Adult, and natural (free) and adapted Child.

Games: Since the publication of Berne's *Games People Play*, the term games has been used and misused in songs, stories, books, and general conversations all over the world. Berne expanded his own definition of games in each book he wrote, and since then transactional analysts have devised widely differing ways of defining and dealing with games. Basically, games are repetitive interactions that end unhappily.

Injunctions and Decisions: Berne believed that the injunction is an all-powerful directive and the decision is an automatic response to the injunction. In his last public speech before his death, Berne told therapists at the Golden Gate Group Therapy Society annual conference, June 1970, "If you have permission to be a winner from your parents, you can cure patients." Traditional transactional analysts continue to write that children are "scripted" by injunctions and counter-injunctions.

Scripts: People develop scripts from injunctions and decisions, which they reinforce throughout their lives by the way they give and receive strokes, the games they play, the partners and friends they choose, and how they interpret life events. The idea of life scripts is now in the public domain. People who have never heard of transactional analysis are discussing their own scripts in conversations, therapy, and support groups.

Strokes: This concept is also so widely used as to be almost banal. Usually lay people refer only to positive strokes when they use the word. Strokes are defined as positive and negative; conditional (for doing) and unconditional (for being); physical (hugs, slaps, etc.), nonverbal (frowns, smiles, etc.), and verbal.

I'm OK—You're OK: This philosophical stance is understood everywhere. It means that all human beings are intrinsically and equally valuable. I'm not OK—You're OK is the depressed position; I'm OK—You're not OK is the paranoid position; I'm not OK—You're not OK is the hopeless position.

Transactional Analysis Practice

Contracts: Transactional analysts and redecision therapists use therapeutic contracts, as originated by Eric Berne. A contract is the specific goal of each individual's therapy, decided by the client with the support of the therapist. In the 1960s and 70s the concept of client contracts was a radical innovation. Prior to that time, the therapist diagnosed the client and made treatment goals without sharing them with the patient. Clinics and hospitals had "case conferences," to which the client was never invited, to decide what the client's goals should be. Contractual psychotherapy truly gave the power back to the client, as client and therapist collaborated on pragmatic diagnoses as well as treatment goals.

Group therapy: This was the favored modality. Eric Berne listened to group interactions and then he and the therapy group analyzed ego states, transactions, games, injunctions, and scripts. He believed strongly in cure through the therapist's "bull's eye" (accurate explanation or confrontation in very few, cogent words that the patient would accept in all ego states.) He believed that potency, permission to change and protection while changing were attributes of the therapist.

Redecision Theory and Practice

Contracts: Redecision work begins with the client contract, just as in classical transactional analysis. Bob Goulding was famous for beginning a piece of work with the question, "What are you going to change about yourself today?" We believed that it was important for clients to claim their own potency, give themselves permission to change, and learn to protect themselves.

Autonomy: People are in charge of our their emotions, thoughts, and behavior. This stance is basic in redecision therapy. To believe that others make us feel, think, or act is to be a victim. To believe we have the power to control the emotions, thoughts, and actions of others, makes us either ineffectual rescuers or perpetual persecutors. Many transactional analysts continue to believe that people's feelings are dependent on the behavior of those around them. They ask, "How does that make you feel?" rather than "How do you feel about that?" The difference between the two questions is crucial in therapy. This does not negate the necessity for human beings to be kind and caring toward each other.

Strokes: We believe in the power of positive stroking and work to keep negative stroking out of groups. Positive stroking by therapists and group members creates a healthy climate for change. I want every session to end in a victory for a client. If a redecision is not made, then perhaps I will stroke the person for understanding the issue, for clarifying, for daring to address a complicated or humiliating problem, for whatever the person has accomplished. Each person who works always accomplishes something!

Ego States: The client uses all three ego states, especially Adult, to settle on a contract. Therapy is most likely to succeed if the contract is pleasing to the natural (free) Child. To make a redecision the client enters a scene as an adapted Child and makes a free Child redecision within the scene. Both Adult and a positive internal Parent support the redecision.

Games: Redecision therapists tend to differ from other transactional analysts in their use of game theory and practice. There are times when we analyze games in the classical manner, using ego state circles and transactional lines. We may show a client Karpman's triangle (persecutor, rescuer, and victim) and diagram how the players change roles during the game. Therapy group members may suggest alternatives to games.

Bob Goulding developed our definition of games:

1. A game begins with what seems to be an Adult stimulus.
2. Within this stimulus is a secret message from Parent or Child.
3. The responder responds to the secret message rather than to the Adult stimulus.
4. The game ends with a pay-off that includes an unhappy emotion plus specific beliefs about self, others, and perhaps fate.
5. The sequence of the game (1 - 4) is not within the conscious awareness of the players.

Games can be complicated or very simple, harmless or dangerous, depending on the game and the players.

Petar is a young physician who is unhappy with his wife. 1. On Saturday mornings Petar can expect to hear, "Petar, the grass needs mowing." 2. This may seem to be an Adult observation but it actually is a Parent command: cut the grass. 3. Petar argues from his adapted (rebellious) Child that the grass can't need cutting so soon, that he has an important engagement, and that he'll try to do it later in the week. They argue back and forth during the rest of the week. Eventually, Petar mows the grass. 4. Payoff: Petar is angry and says to himself, "She cares nothing about what I want" and "I never have any fun in this marriage."

In our method of working with games, we focus on the payoff, which is often a repetition of childhood decisions about self and others. I suggest to Petar, "Close your eyes, experience your anger, and say to yourself, 'Nobody cares what I want' and 'I can't have any fun in life.' Is there a scene in your childhood that fits your anger and your words?"

Petar responds with fury, "That's all there's ever been in my life!" He reenacts a scene in which he is at home studying. He can hear his friends playing outside and wants to join them, but his father is forcing Petar to study instead of play. In fantasy he expresses to his father his anger and then somewhat reluctantly he acknowledges that his father's pressure is helping him get the grades he needs to be accepted in medical school. He tells his father, "You are right, but so am I. I should have time for play."

He comes back to the present. "Damn! What am I doing mowing my own lawn! Now I'm the one not letting me play." He brings his father and his wife into a present-day fantasy and tells them, "I am never mowing the lawn again. I am a physician. I am spending my money hiring kids to mow my lawn. If this bothers either of you, see a therapist!"

Injunctions, Decisions, and Redecisions: We believe that an injunction is given by a parental figure and sometimes by the clients themselves. A Parental injunction is not automatically accepted, as Berne believed. The acceptance of an injunction constitutes the decision. A redecision is a change in thoughts, emotions, beliefs, and/or actions that counteract a decision. It is the freeing of oneself from the restraints of the decision. A redecision is made within a reenacted scene from childhood (as in Petar's scene), the recent past, a dream, an imaginary scene, or the present. After a redecision is made, clients need to practice their changes in the present, as Petar will do when he hires someone to mow his lawn.

As an example of redecision therapy I will use my work with a patient, described in my article, "The Joy of Therapy."

A depressed woman in a five-day workshop says, "I want to decide to live." From the contract and clarification work of the two previous days, I know her diagnosis, her current difficulties, and her early decisions. Now comes the vital work. I am already excited. "OK, what scene do you want to use?" I am suggesting that she will be successful using any scene she picks. I want her to breathe in my confidence.

"I don't know. Whatever scene you pick."

I'd love to think for her, if only that were wise. I love to plan scenes. "Hey, you know yourself better than I'll ever know you. You are ready to decide not to kill yourself ... to live. What scene?"

Silence and sighs. "I don't know if I know how to do this."

I must remember that she wants to be successful even more than I want it for her, but she has only herself to bring to this important moment. I have her and myself and hundreds of other people who have decided to live in this very room. "Take your time."

She goes limp, waiting. Maybe we'll have to deal first with her passivity, her transference. I invent here and now scenes, but don't want to use them. I wonder how many thousand scenes I have invented and not used. "What scene did you think of and cross out?"

"They used to put me in the cellar when I wouldn't eat." She describes the cellar, the horror of it.

"Be there." I don't want to keep her too long in that cellar. Sometimes the re-living of past pain produces drama for the therapist and group members, and a sense of psychological rape in the victim. "Tell your parents you won't kill yourself in spite of what they are doing to you."

She does, and we work together as she affirms her decision to live. Then she says, "I don't feel it. That was just an exercise."

Oh, damn. I feel a split-second frustration-twinge of countertransference, but also know I moved her too quickly. "That's OK. You found an important scene." I run through possible options in my head. Then, "You said yesterday that last month you were very suicidal. You made plans to kill yourself." I am talking and at the same time feeling her despair and her characteristic helplessness. "This time... be in your home when you are considering suicide. OK?"

"Yes. I thought about it a lot."

A few more questions and she is in her living room a month ago, planning her suicide in detail. While she talks, I hear key words only, and am searching for the best way for her to end triumphantly.

"In spite of your plans, some part of you kept you from murdering you." I set up two chairs, not facing each other. "Sit here and be the part of you that does not want to kill you, that doesn't want to go along with murder." She doesn't know how to start, so I have her change to the self-murderer chair. "Be the part of you who wants to murder you."

She does this, replaying briefly what she said about wanting to die.

"Now, change chairs. Be the part of you who says no."

"I guess I don't want to end everything."

"Say it without 'I guess.'"

"I don't want to end everything. Life is an adventure."

Wow! So easy. She just came right out with it. Now there is no question where to go. Now being in the cellar is necessary pain. "Be back in the cellar, really be there, and know that you do not want to end everything. Say, "I don't want to end everything. My life is an adventure." I think I'm talking softly. Silently I'm saying, Don't blow it! You've almost won! "You're in the cellar. Stand up and say it ..."

She leaps to her feet, crying and shouting, "I don't want to end everything. I'm smashing the door! That's what I'm doing. I'm smashing the door! I'm out! I'm out of the cellar!" She sits down, smiling and a little dazed. "I'm not killing myself." After a few moments she goes on, explaining to herself what she has just learned ... that she'd always been psychologically in that cellar and hadn't known it. She says she's free. She shakes her head. "I can hardly believe it. It was the cellar. I didn't know." She smiles. "I did it."

During a later session she discusses how to arrange her life so that it is an adventure, as well as how to keep herself alive during periods when she can't find adventure.

Redecision therapy is an interweaving of a client's and therapist's fantasies. It is the creating of imaginary scenes that unfold almost simultaneously in the minds of client and therapist. The resolution of these imaginary scenes is the redecision. To be effective a redecision therapist needs imagination, playfulness, and the ability to be a part of the client's world, both real and imaginary. Humor is a plus, as is love of theater. The therapist may demonstrate the quickness of a stand-up comedian. Most important is the therapist's absolute belief in the client. The therapy may seem magical but, as Bob Goulding said, "There is no 'magic' in redecision work." Like juggling or magic tricks, good redecision therapy is learned. It is learned by therapists willing to develop and enhance their own Child and listen to the

Child in their clients.

What has redecision therapy given to transactional analysis? A lightness of touch and an emphasis on the emotional realities of an individual life. A belief that the power to effect change truly resides in the patient, even though it also resides in the ability of the therapist to aid in the process. It is child-like, visual, visceral, emotional, spontaneous. Although clients may forget much of what occurs in therapy, they will remember for years a single scene in which they moved from victim to victor. We redecision therapists give to Transactional Analysis a sense of personal autonomy and the proof that the Child in each of us can be energized, expanded, enriched ... and that this process does change lives.

References

1. Eric Berne's books are again in print and available.
2. Eric Berne, MD, "Away From A Theory Of The Impact Of Interpersonal Interaction On Non-Verbal Participation", *Transactional Analysis Journal,* 1:1, January 1971.
3. Mary Goulding, "What Transactional Analysis and Redecision Therapy Gave Each Other," *Redecision Journal*, Vol. 1, No.14.
4. Mary Goulding, "The Joy Of Psychotherapy," p 4-7 Leslie B. Kadis, MD, editor, *Redecision Therapy: Expanded Perspectives,*1985.
5. *Transactional Analysis Journals*, collected and reprinted by the International Transactional Analysis Association

TWO

A Redecision Workshop*

*Some of this material was first published in *Redecision Therapy* journal.

For many years I have taught redecision therapy in workshops in the United States and abroad. Here is a format for a five-day workshop. It can also be used effectively as two or three weekend workshops. It combines brief lectures, demonstrations, and practice by the participants. I believe practice is most important and can be done effectively in triads, because each person then has the opportunity to use redecision techniques without the anxiety of being watched by the whole group. The following workshop is an amalgam of several recent workshops.

1. FIRST DAY, morning

Introductions.

I explain the general format: lecture, demonstration, therapy in triads, discussion, plus one afternoon for help with any problems regarding clients or patients in their own practices. Each day the triads will change.

Lecture. **Contracts for personal change.** All redecision work is based on personal, very specific contracts for change. The change may be in behavior, emotions, beliefs, and/or self-concept. It must be understandable to both therapist and client, be achievable, beneficial to the client and not harmful to others. I explain the difference between "should" (Parent) and "want" (Child) contracts. I discuss the importance of "no suicide" and "no homicide" contracts, which take precedence over all other contracts. Next in importance are contracts specifying "no abuse of self or others."

There are times when the contract is self-evident and I'll spend only a minute or two discussing it with the client; for example, a contract to stop being afraid of spiders. Sometimes a contract may be to "explore": "I have three job offers and want to explore my thoughts and feelings before deciding what to do." Sometimes the contract is to recover from a trauma or loss.

Demonstration. John states that he wants to stop sabotaging himself on the job. I ask him to recall a recent scene in which he does what he calls "sabotaging myself on the job." "Be in that scene, and tell it in the present tense as if it were actually happening right now." He plays himself and his director, Dr. Reeves. I stop him from time to time for clarification or to ask what he is feeling. In the scene the director is asking John about his work and John becomes flustered and defensive. He concludes, "I want to react with Dr. Reeves the way I do with my clients. I am not defensive with them."

Lecture. **Autonomy.** No one can control our thoughts, our emotions, or our actions. We are in charge of ourselves. Those who do not recognize this are often unsuccessful in reaching their goals, because they blame others for their problems. They want others to change before they are willing to change themselves. We will be emphasizing autonomy throughout this workshop.

Break

Practice. The group divides itself into triads to establish **contracts.** One person will be therapist, one will be client, and one will be both observer and co-therapist if the therapist asks for help. The observer will note aloud if the client or therapist talks about an issue rather than experiencing it in the here and now. The observer will also look for non-autonomous language, such as "he made me feel," "I suppose I can try," or "it just happened." When the contract has been established, the members of the triad will change roles until each person has had the opportunity to make a contract. When they have finished, participants report their experiences to the whole group and announce their contracts.

Lecture. **Free and Adapted Child in Redecision Therapy.** A Free Child is not under the influence of either an external or internal Parent. An Adapted Child is or was under the influence of a Parent. The adaptation may be a decision made in order to be loved or to be protected against real or imagined dangers. These decisions are responses to injunctions, traumas, or personal genetic or biological traits. I explain the list of injunctions that Bob Goulding and I developed: Don't exist, Don't do, Don't feel, Don't think, Don't grow, Don't be successful, Don't be a child, Don't trust, Don't love, Don't be sexual, Don't belong, Don't want or need, Don't be well or sane, Don't be who you are. A decision is like an emotional or intellectual straitjacket and a redecision, made by the Free Child, is the removal of the straitjacket. A redecision brings new freedom, new ways to think, feel, or act. Positive Parenting supports the redecision. During the week, I will demonstrate various ways of doing redecision therapy.

Practice. Introducing the Free Child. In the triads I ask the participants to go back in time to a young age and remember themselves playing happily. What is the child doing? Watch and enjoy this child. Experience this child as unique and lovable. Then introduce the child proudly to your colleagues. "I want you to meet young ______, whom I love very much." If for any reason anyone has difficulty with this exercise, the other two in the triad will help.

The Adapted Child can be compliant (obedient), rebellious, or withdrawn. The compliant Child wants to be accepted. Remember yourself sitting in church or trying to impress the grownups at your parents' cocktail party or being "good" in school. The rebellious Child fights back, doing the opposite of what the grownups want. The withdrawn Child daydreams and doesn't listen. You may choose to remember a scene in which you accepted or lived out one of the injunctions. Introduce this child to your triad.

2. FIRST DAY, afternoon

Lecture. **Client Strengths.** Too often psychotherapy is based on pathology, on what is wrong with the client. It is more important to know what is right with the client. What are the client's strengths?

Practice. Go back to childhood in fantasy and remember your own strengths. Find three specific child strengths and remember a scene that highlights at least one of them. Be the age you are when the scene occurs and relive the scene in the triad. Afterwards, discuss how the use of your childhood strengths might facilitate achieving your contract. Some participants may volunteer to tell their scenes to the entire group. Here are examples:

"I am six years old and I collect pretty pebbles from driveways and arrange them into families. Families have troubles. Children get lost or get sick. Sometimes somebody dies and I set up a funeral and bury the stone. Sometimes they have birthday parties. The children go to school and I am the teacher. When I find new stones, they become new families who move into the neighborhood. If I have a family I am tired of, I pretend they move away. It is exciting to manage a whole town full of people. Strengths: imagination, ability to manage a whole imaginary town, excitement. Oh, yes, also independence. I don't need other people to entertain me."

"I am eight years old during the Spanish Civil War. We are Communists and when the Fascists arrive in our town, my father is shot, killed. My mother, my little sister, and I have no way to get food. I happen to find a stack of cardboard by an abandoned shed. I drag it home and cut it up to make toys. I make wagons with wheels that turn and dolls whose arms and legs move, and other things. I take the toys around the village and trade them for food for my family. My toys keep my family alive. My strengths are determination, ability to solve problems, and I made good toys."

"My asset is humor. At the dinner table, my father gets angry at somebody and starts yelling. I tremble and twitch and act super scared, and he knows I am just play acting and he starts laughing. At school, when a teacher is upset at me over some little thing, I say, 'That is probably the worst, most disgusting thing I have ever done in my entire life,' and the way I say it gets her laughing. My real asset is I've always been a cheery sort. Drives some people nuts. But mostly people like me. I am also astute in sizing up people."

Demonstration. I offer to be therapist for someone who wants to use Child strengths to fulfill a contract. One client is literally bouncing in her chair as she volunteers. "I thought this was going to be long, hard, painful work. My contract is to say goodbye to my lover. I mean, we were lovers and I hoped we'd get married and always be together, but we were only together two months and that was two years ago. I keep trying to get him back. I've suffered terribly about this. My strength in my story is my ability to empathize and to be sensitive. I do understand his feelings and mine, and I suffer. My feelings are so damned precious." She explains that her lover wanted fun, not a commitment. "He is into romance, not into an enduring relationship. I hurt and analyze my hurt over and over."

Again she is bouncing and giggling. "But now ... well, screw empathy and sensitivity. When I heard Pete tell about at school how he told the teacher it was the worst thing he had ever done .. all that stuff ... and how he could get people laughing ... THAT'S WHAT I NEED! THAT'S WHAT I REALLY NEED! A HUMOROUS CHILD!" She jumps off her chair and walks around the room, pulling her hair and pretending to sob, as she makes a huge drama out of losing her lover and never being happy again. The group laughs and applauds.

When she is finished, she says, "And to think I spent all this money to come here to suffer more about me and my lover, and now I've solved everything in five minutes. Do I get a refund?" She laughs again. "Refund or not, I won't suffer."

(Sometimes a therapist's job is amazingly easy. I only had to listen.)

Practice. In the triads, one person is therapist, one observer or co-therapist, and one client. The clients will use their own Child strengths or borrowed strengths to fulfill their contracts. Each triad will do only one piece of work.

Break

Discussion. Participants report successes or problems encountered during the therapy work. I am available to work briefly with anyone who was a client and wasn't satisfied with the result.

Lecture. The **Positive Parent** is sometimes nurturing, sometimes restrictive (don't hit your brother!) but always on the side of growth. We learn to love from being loved. We learn to nurture from being nurtured.

Practice. Participants return again in fantasy to their childhood and this time remember a scene in which some parent or parent figure is instrumental in changing their lives positively. In the triads, they tell their scenes. I ask if anyone would like to share with the whole group.

"My parents are very austere types, who don't praise. But my grandmother holds me and calls me her 'darlingest, prettiest little love.' I think I learned from her that I am lovable. My contract is to ... well ... like myself. I am going to keep remembering her."

"In high school my English teacher asks the students who plan to go to college to raise their hands. I don't, because no one in my family ever went to college. The teacher says, 'Robert, you raise your hand right now! You are smart enough to go to college and you must go! It would be criminal to cheat yourself out of a college education!' Her statement changed my life."

Lecture. **Strokes.** Strokes are positive or negative; physical, nonverbal, or verbal; for being (I love/hate you because you exist) or for doing (I love/hate what you did.)

Practice. Participants are asked if there are important Parent strokes they have wanted and lacked. One at a time they ask for these strokes from the other members of their triad. Participants receive these specific, desired Parental strokes. Next, participants imagine themselves holding the child on their laps, and giving the child the strokes they have just received. In this way, participants begin the process of self-reparenting.

Members of each triad say good-bye for today to members of their triad and give each other whatever positive feedback they choose. Tomorrow participants will be in different triads.

3. SECOND DAY, morning

Discussion and brags. Each morning clients are encouraged to brag about anything they have learned or experienced in the course of the workshop. This is followed by a brief question period covering yesterday's work. I announce that we will spend the morning on Redecision therapy and in the afternoon I'll finish with ego states by dealing with the negative Parent.

Demonstration. I ask for a volunteer who already is aware of an early scene that fits his or her contract. I will do redecision work, using the scene the volunteer selects.

Fred volunteers. "I do have an early scene. But I don't know if there is anything I can do about it."

"Let's see. Your contract is?"

"It has to do with being perfect. I'm very hard on myself when I don't do things perfectly."

"Bob Goulding used to remind people that there was only one

person on earth who was perfect, and look what happened to him."

Fred smiles. "I'm not in danger of being perfect. Like ... I'm not perfect but I am very afraid of making a mistake." He explains that while he is in this city to attend this workshop, he has been asked to interview a psychologist who wants to join the mental health group to which he belongs. "I'm afraid of the responsibility. Maybe I'll decide he is fine for our group and he'll turn out not to be. Maybe I'll have reservations about him and really he'd have been what we want. I agonize about this."

"What is your childhood scene?"

He tells of a bleak childhood in Europe after World War II. The family is always hungry, his father has come home crippled from a war injury and can't work. There is no employment anyway. Fred's about eight. His father has given him a bit of money to buy meat for soup for the family.

"Be there. Be eight. OK?"

"I am in a long line, waiting to get the meat. My father has told me to hide the money so no one knows I have it and I put it in my pocket. I think that's where it is but I am afraid to check. I am waiting in line and when I get to the front of the line, I can't find the money. It's gone. I can't believe it. It's not anywhere. The meat man yells at me, 'If you don't have money get out of the line.' Somebody pushes me. I'll never know what happened to the money. I don't know how I could have lost it, but I did. It was a terrible thing to do. Somebody must have gotten it out of my pocket." He is afraid to go home, but finally does. "My father screams at me that I am worthless, and he beats me. He says we're all going to starve to death because of me..."

"Hey, wait. This is too much for an eight year old to handle. Let me be in the house with you, OK? You be Father. Please sit down over there on that chair, Father. I want to talk to you."

Very softly, I say to client-as-father, "Don't hit your son. That won't help. It won't bring the money back. This life is too hard for all of you, isn't it? It must be especially hard for you, hurt from the war, not able to take care of your family the way you want to, having to give the money to a little kid instead of getting the meat yourself. I am sorry you have such a difficult, difficult life."

Client-as-father is crying. I suggest to the client that he go back to his own chair. He sobs for some time.

"Would you be willing, after all this time, to see your father in your mind and to forgive him for not being a perfect father? For making terrible mistakes in his treatment of you?"

Fred is still crying. "I thought I was worthless. I never forgave myself. Forgive my father? That's strange." He tells his father that he understands and he forgives him.

"And now, do you realize that you made no mistake. You have nothing whatsoever to forgive yourself for?"

He listens quietly.

"Everybody in that line was hungry. Some of them had turned into thieves in order to stay alive, right? Somebody in the line got your money. That's all. It's over."

"It wasn't my fault. It's over. It is over."

Later he says, "About the psychologist. He'll be an asset to the team or he won't be. Whatever, no one is going to starve."

Discussion. I answer questions about techniques. As in all pieces of work, there were options. Sometimes it is better to focus on unexpressed emotions. To do that I might have questioned more about what he was feeling in line and at home. If he had a problem expressing anger and that was part of his contract, then I might have had him beat on pillows and yell his anger at his father before forgiving his father and himself. Or I might have had him enter the scene as the adult, instead of my entering it. As an adult, he'd tell young Fred that he'll protect him from now on and give Fred permission to make mistakes.

Practice. The group forms into new triads. In each triad one person will be therapist, one co-therapist or observer, and one will be a client who remembers a relevant early scene that seems to fit the contract. There will be time for only one piece of redecision work in each triad.

Discussion. Each triad presents its work and the members stroke each other for what was accomplished. One triad said they were stuck, so I offered to work briefly with the client. Nancy considers her distrust of men to be related to her father's abandoning her family when she was a child. The therapist did a good job, working with her in a scene with father, but Nancy wants to change the reality of the scene in order for father to ask her forgiveness.

Demonstration. I wonder aloud how it would help Nancy trust other men to pretend father was solicitous when he wasn't. Wouldn't that simply emphasize that father was not to be trusted?

Nancy: "I suppose so. But I want him to change."

"So tell him that."

She does, tearfully.

"Now tell him that you want him to change back then, when you are a little girl."

"I want you to change ... But that's impossible."

"Exactly. You are saying you are not going to trust any man today until your father changes when you are a little girl."

"So it's all hopeless."

"Trying to change the past is hopeless. You can understand the past in a new way or imagine changing yourself in the past." I congratulate her and her group on understanding her impasse and suggest she work again tomorrow. To the group, I say that many of their clients are not changing today because they are waiting for the past to change. One of the most important aspects in therapy is saying good-bye to a long gone past.

Break

Lecture. **Negative Parents.** There are three types of negative parenting. One is the Over-nurturing Parent, who does for the child what it is healthier for the child to do. This Parent keeps the child helpless and unsure of his or her own abilities. The injunctions imposed by the Over-nurturing Parent are "Don't grow," "Don't think," and "Don't do."

Another negative parent is the Critical Parent. This is the one that transactional analysts are most likely to focus on, inasmuch as it is the Parent who often blocks therapy. This Parent also may cause considerable personal pain and shame, telling you that you are no good, not good enough, or that what you said was silly or incorrect. This Parent may have been a real parent, an older sibling, or the type of teacher who marks all of your mistakes in bright red but doesn't give you positive strokes.

Practice. This time we will work in the large group. I ask all participants to remember a recent time when they were being self-critical. Maybe you misplaced your glasses or your wallet, were crabby to your children, or were late to a meeting. What does this Critical Parent say to you? I ask if everyone has found a self-critical statement. When all have, I suggest everyone stand up and do an "awkward dance" while loudly criticizing self. I show them how by standing up, dancing awkwardly, and screeching, "How could you have done that AGAIN!" Everyone stands up, dances, yells, and laughs.

Then I show them how to criticize themselves with the accent on the wrong syllàble, lisping, or squeaking like a pig, and again the group practices all at the same time.

There are many more ways of getting rid of the Critical parent. I suggest: imagine the Parent in your head as a witch, ogre, or clown, put that Parent on your TV screen, watch and listen until you are bored, and then change channels to a sex or adventure channel. It is also fun to send this Parent on a spaceship to Mars. An assignment for tomorrow is to find other ways of making fun of or removing the Critical Parent.

Lecture. The third type of negative parent is the Prejudiced Parent, which you may have incorporated from society, your culture, religious and governmental leaders, as well as from actual parents. Examples are racial, religious, and sexual bigotry. People are victimized by the terrible combination of what Eric Berne called the fascist in the Child coupled with the Prejudiced Parent.

Practice. Close your eyes and remember an early scene in which you were either a victim or a persecutor because of prejudice. Perhaps your remembered scene is your first encounter with someone who is of a different race, sexual orientation, or religion. Perhaps you were humiliated because you were poor, so didn't have the right clothes to wear to school. Share stories in your triad. If you want to forgive yourself or another or want to say goodbye to that scene, ask for help from your triad. Some participants report their successes to the large group.

4. SECOND DAY, afternoon

Lecture. **Emotions.** Emotional health is the ability to feel all feelings, to express them orally and with appropriate body language, to use them for appropriate actions, and then to let the feelings subside. Anger is shown by scowls, often a loud voice, and clenched fists. Smiles or tears or placating gestures are inappropriate when a person is expressing anger. Sadness may be expressed in a softer voice and often with tears. Scowls, loudness, and smiles are inappropriate when expressing sadness. Often children are confused when their parents smile as they speak angrily or show anger when they are actually sad. They are confused if their parents deny feelings when their voice tones, gestures, and facial expression tell a child that the adult is sad, angry, frightened, or embarrassed.

Who in your family was the angry one? Who was sad, fearful, worried, guilty, excited, enthusiastic, calm? Who didn't show feelings at all?

1. Children copy their parents' chronic emotions.
2. Children get strokes for expressing certain emotions. Some children are cuddled and kissed when they are sad and ignored when they are happy; others, particularly boys, get positive recognition for being angry.
3. Children learn to repress emotions that are dangerous in their families. A child may be punished for crying or may be frightened because a parent overreacts to anger. When a child represses a feeling, that child usually covers it with another. When anger is dangerous, the child expresses sadness instead. When sadness is dangerous, anger may be used to cover sadness.

Demonstration. I ask for a volunteer to demonstrate a feeling response from TV or real life. Annie plays out a scene in which a neighbor is furious because a workman did a poor job of building her fence. Then other volunteers tell the same story, using sadness, anxiety, or humor.

Practice. In triads participants practice showing their feelings authentically. They also practice using feelings they usually suppress.

Break

Demonstration. I do redecision therapy with volunteers for the rest of the afternoon.

5. THIRD DAY, morning

Discussion, brags, questions, and comments. Some bring new, silly ways to deal with the Critical Parent. I announce that I will work with one or two clients, and then the group will form new triads for redecision work. In the afternoon we will explore Games.

Demonstration. **Redecision using family sculpture,** which I first learned from Virginia Satir. Nancy wants to finish yesterday's work. If she is willing, I think it will be interesting for her to do a sculpture of her family just before her father leaves the family. She is intrigued. I tell her, "Pick people from the group to represent your father, mother, brothers and sisters, anyone else in the family at that time, and yourself." She is six, her brother is ten, and her sister is nine. She adds, "There is an important person I never met, the woman my father is running off to marry." She asks a participant to be that woman.

"Sculpt each person to show how that person fits into the family. Start with father and mother and the "other woman," putting them at the distance from each other that seems right to you." She does, putting father closer to the "other woman" than to his wife. "Now put the children in the sculpture wherever you think they fit. Move their arms and hands, legs, heads, faces to show their emotions. Or demonstrate a posture and facial expression so that the person can copy you."

Nancy sculpts her mother with a fist raised toward father and her other hand beside her eyes to show she is crying. Father has one hand blocking himself from his family and is reaching for the "other woman." Brother stands beside mother, and has both fists raised against father. Sister is alone, looking off in the distance, hands on hips, paying attention to no one. Nancy sculpts the person representing herself as running from mother to father and back, with her arms held up as if she is a baby pleading to be held. She takes her own place in the sculpture and begins to cry. She says, "This is so sad." I ask her to tell each family member that, and then say something else to each one. To father, "I am so sad. Please don't go." To mother "I am so sad. Make him stay." To brother: "Stop fighting Daddy and make him stay." To sister: "You never cared about anybody."

"What do you feel when no one responds to you?"

Nancy sobs, "More and more sad."

"Keep moving from father to mother and back. Imagine the years passing, year after year, and you are still running back and forth, holding up your arms as you try to get them to change." She does this, and makes no move on her own toward resolution. I ask the rest of the men in the workshop to stand up, walk around the scene, and wave and smile at Nancy.

"The years are going by and many men smile and wave at you, but you are too busy crying for your father. You don't let yourself see the other men in the world."

The men keep walking, the family stays in the sculpture, and I ask if she is going to do anything or if she is going to spend the rest of her life in this one scene.

"Maybe I should get out of this mess." She walks slowly away from her family. She still appears very sad.

"Maybe, or maybe you should stay in it. Your choice."

"Damn, damn, damn!" Her tears are gone, and she looks angry. "But what if all men are just like my father?"

I say, "If you try very very hard, you can probably find one as untrustworthy for you as he was."

She glares at me, then smiles. "OK. I get it. I'm done. Thank you."

I ask each member of the sculpture to give feedback.

Later in the workshop she does more work, deciding what she will want to change about herself in order to seek out healthy, loving men. First, of course, she needs to esteem herself.

Demonstration. I decide to demonstrate another way of doing family sculpture. James' contract is to claim his own importance at home and at work. I ask group members to help him bring a table from the back of the room to the center. James seats his family of origin around this dinner table. Father is at the head and mother at the foot. although she is so busy serving food that she rarely sits. Three brothers are on one side. He and his two sisters are on the other. I ask who is important at the family meal. "Only father." Father leads them in prayer and then pontificates about his day. One brother talks about his baseball game but no one listens. Mother talks only to urge the youngest to eat more.

I say, "What a boring meal! How can you stir things up?"

James says, "I don't know. Nobody will listen."

"You want to be important. Be important."

"It's not possible."

"Bet you a nickel."

He grins. "Hey, all of you. I am important."

(I tell the others not to respond.)

He sighs, then says loudly, "Hey, I know what is wrong with this family. NOBODY IS IMPORTANT. That's the truth. Dad, you are boring. Mother, you are boring. We are all boring. I need to learn how to be interesting if I want to feel important." He thinks a moment. "We need to learn how to be interested in each other. I am going to be interested in my brother's ball games. He asks about the ball game. Then, spontaneously, "Hey, all of you, do you know I am building my own racer out of orange crates and real wheels! I've almost got it done and it's beautiful and complicated but I never talk about it because I haven't known how to interest you." He tells them about his orange crate racer.

James asks if he can substitute his current family for the old one, and does. He sits down with the participants who represent his wife and two sons. "I used to preach at you. Not church stuff, but equally preachy. I learned it from my father. And now you are all in terrible danger of ending up unimportant bores like I have been." He tells them a joke he learned at the workshop. "From now on, we are all going to be interested and interesting."

He tells the group, "I'm going to have to put a lot of effort into this. I think I am understanding how to do it and I am going to practice being interesting here at the workshop. While I practice, I'd like your comments."

I suggest that he ask for support rather than comments, and that he is important enough to choose what is helpful.

Lecture. I describe possible uses of family sculpture, such as having each family member in family therapy sculpt the family as he or she sees it and then talk about their perspectives. In working with businesses, a therapist can suggest that each participant sculpt the major problem as each sees it. In any sculpture, the client may take the place of others in the sculpture to understand them better. Sometimes I interview various members of a sculpture. Clients may sculpt their dreams.

Break.

Practice. Participants do family sculpture in groups of six or nine.

6. THIRD DAY, afternoon

Lecture. **Redecision Therapy and Games.** Games are stereotyped interactions that end in mutual unhappiness. What happens over and over again at your house, at your business, or among your friends that ends up with unhappiness? How does it start? What happens next? And next? How does it end?

Practice. Participants close their eyes and imagine themselves in their past or current homes. If they prefer, they can imagine themselves at work or with friends. In triads participants tell their games in the present tense. When the game is over, "*What do you feel in one word* and what do you secretly say *about yourself, the others,* and perhaps *what do you say about fate?*" After telling their games in the triads, some volunteer to tell them to the entire group:

"Mother is late getting ready for an outing... wherever we go... and everyone is pushing her to hurry up. She gets mad. The rest of us are unhappy. *I am frustrated* and say to myself *'there is nothing I can do'* and *'she doesn't really care about what is important to us.'*"

"Father tells us not to worry, he can fix the car. But he can't. Finally, after a week of not having a car, it gets towed to the garage. *I am anxious* and say *'He is incompetent. We are both incompetent.'*"

"My daughter borrows my blouse without asking and returns it with a spot on it. *I am furious.* I say, *'she is totally inconsiderate in spite of all the nice things I do for her.'"*

"The Boss finds a minor mistake made by one of us and exaggerates it. The one he is criticizing looks very sad and embarrassed. The rest of us rescue the sad one by saying that the mistake is not the least bit important and is easily corrected. Now the boss is sad and talks about team loyalty. Pretty soon everyone is angry. *'I am angry and frustrated. I wish I had the nerve to leave this job.'"*

A participant reminds the group of a game played before dinner last night. "Someone says 'I don't know what to do about my son.' Several of us give suggestions and she argues against every suggestion. *I am frustrated.* I say to myself, *'I tried to help but she doesn't listen.'"*

My group and I have already solved my game! The game is, "I ask my husband if he will clean up the garage, which he keeps a total mess. He says he will, but he doesn't. We argue, he promises, he does nothing, and I end up depressed. Sad. I say to myself, *'I try so hard and do so many things for him and he doesn't care about me. He doesn't love me.'"* My group asked me if I have any examples of the way he does love me. And whether he is more important than his garbage. I decide that I will go home and tell him I love him and I know he loves me, and from now on the garage belongs to him. I won't even look in it. I am happy. I feel as if a huge weight is off my back.

Break

Lecture. I give several options for solving games. 1. Change your usual feelings or behavior during the game or immediately after it is over. 2. Stop playing as soon as you recognize the game and give yourself lots of positive strokes for doing this. 3. Practice crossing transactions, stroking positively instead of criticizing, for example. Or be factual instead of emotional. 4. Recognize your stereotyped role in games. Are you usually a persecutor, rescuer, or victim? Switch roles and exaggerate to make your switch humorous. 5. Primarily in redecision therapy we use the payoff, the negative feeling plus the statements of self and others, as a way of reaching back to early child decisions.

Demonstration. The woman whose daughter borrows her clothes has fun pretending to sob and be a classical victim. Then she acts out being a screaming, threatening persecutor. Finally she is a whiny rescuer who says she knows her poor daughter didn't mean to soil her blouse. When she finishes, she decides she will simply stop the game. She tells her daughter firmly that she will no longer permit her to borrow clothing.

The person who asked for help with her son uses her own payoff to go back to an early scene. She leaves hopelessness behind, in her childhood scene. She was hopeless then, but not now. She figures out for herself what she is going to do to solve her problem with her son.

Practice. In triads, the participants work with each other to stop their games, and then report.

7. FOURTH DAY, morning

Brags, questions, and discussion.

Demonstration. John, the man I worked with during the contract-setting stage, wants to work with me. His contract is to stop sabotaging himself on the job. He says he has learned a great deal in just three days. He is giving and accepting positive strokes, for example. But he is still worried about how he will deal with his director. "I just somehow stop thinking when I am with him. It's... you know... no, I know... I'll always say something wrong."

"Put your director in the chair opposite you and tell him this."

"I don't really like doing this."

"Say to your director, I don't like doing this."

"Well, the fact is, I am supposed to, well, talk to you, Dr. Reeves, and I don't like saying this to you ... well, I don't want you to know... you know... well, I am always nervous around you. Somehow, I always end up in the wrong. I don't think you like dealing with me either..."

"Skip that part for now. For now, repeat in your head, 'Somehow I will end up in the wrong,' and see how that fits in your past."

John looks startled. "It's like with my brother. It's hard to believe ... they really aren't at all alike. My brother really... well ... is not very intelligent. But, yes, it's my brother. My brother always knew all the answers. He didn't like me. He always made me wrong."

John is holding his arms tightly over his chest, as if to protect himself.

I could work with his rigidly defensive, almost frightened posture, but instead have a hunch I decide to use. "How old was your brother when you were born?"

"Carl is three years older than me."

"I'll bet he wasn't very happy about you coming into his life."

"My parents joke about his telling them to take me back to the hospital."

"My hunch is that he spent his childhood proving he was better than you."

John nods. "He could do it, too."

"Not really better, but it seemed that way to you. You learn to walk and he's already been walking for three years. You learn to read and he already reads. You come home with something, anything, you are excited to have learned and he already knows it. Tough for a little guy like you, John."

"I didn't think of it that way. But that is how it was." John is smiling now. "I knew I wasn't dumb, just like I know that with Dr. Reeves, but I always manage to seem dumb."

"Yeah. You were not dumb. You just had a jealous older brother. Bring up another chair for your brother. Right there next to Dr. Reeves. Now really see the two of them, Carl and Dr. Reeves. See the differences between them"

John sees several differences. His director is not jealous of him, is more intelligent than Carl. Then John notes the stunning difference. "Dr. Reeves wants me to succeed. That's the difference. That's the real difference!" He now believes he can listen to his director and can tell him honestly when he needs help, rather than try to bluff his way through.

"My guess is that it would be a relief for both of you."

John jumps up and gives me a hug. "Did you notice," he asks, "that I have just done a good piece of work and I listened to both of us?"

Discussion. Some participants relate similar stories during their childhood, either as younger or older child in the family.

Lecture. **Goodbyes.** I discuss the need for goodbyes when a client is not moving forward or remains depressed over a loss. This is particularly necessary for older people, simply because they have lost so much and are not anticipating new adventures in the future. However, it is important for people of any age who seem to have their energy or zest for life bound up in the past. I mention typical instances when goodbyes may be appropriate: death; divorce; lost jobs, homes, physical health, money. I tell of a woman who said goodbye to the joys of high school and being prom queen ... in order to have her energy available for the not-so-glamorous jobs of being a mother and a secretary.

Demonstration. I ask if there is anyone who wants to say a goodbye. A woman explains that two years ago she and her husband had to relocate from New Jersey to Arizona because he received a very fine job offer there. She had just finished graduate school, so was not giving up a job of her own. She is still unhappy with the move, even though she now has a good job in Arizona.

I suggest she be a tour guide and introduce us to her old area, her town, and her home. She does. Then I ask if there is a special place she would like to be as she says goodbye. She chooses to be at the barbecue given in their honor, before they left. "I am with our friends." She tells her friends what she gained from knowing them and living in New Jersey, what she will keep with her in memory from that period in her life, and then tells them what is enriching in her life in Arizona. She says, "I hope you will visit us. I will visit you. But this is a final good-bye. Good-bye, dear home and dear friends." She lets the image of the barbecue fade away.

Discussion and questions.

Break

Lecture. **Trauma.** My technique is to encourage a trauma victim to tell his or her story several times. For example, in dealing with past childhood sexual abuse, it is important first for the patient to understand he or she was not guilty. No child is ever guilty. I suggest the client visit the scene of the abuse, first as a reporter getting the facts, or as his or her adult self. Then the child reenters the scene several times as a child, with her adult self or an imaginary police officer as protector. Each time the child will test out a different emotion. "I am so afraid," "sad," "ashamed," "helpless," "angry." It is important to tell the abuser, "You are evil and you hurt me," and describe the way in which the child was hurt, physically and emotionally. "You took away my innocence." "You damaged my soul." When the child is ready, he or she will end with the knowledge, "I am done with you. I am leaving the past behind. I am whole."

Practice. In triads, the participants will spend the rest of the morning working as therapist and co-therapist, and with any client who was physically or sexually abused in childhood..

8. FOURTH DAY, afternoon

This is the time set aside for whatever the participants want to ask or discuss in terms of their own professional work. They may discuss current clients, office problems, or whatever concerns them. The entire group will discuss and work together on whatever issues emerge.

At the end of the afternoon I will give the group the following fantasy trip: The workshop is over and you are at your home or office. Are there any changes you still want to make in yourself before the workshop is over? Participants report.

9. FIFTH DAY , morning

We skip brags and reports. Those who wish to be clients choose the therapist they prefer and form triads.

Break

Demonstration. I do final, very brief therapy with anyone not finished. If there is no further therapy, we have a question and discussion period.

10. FIFTH DAY, afternoon

The work of the week is finished.

Now is the time for reports and final brags. All participants give specific examples of what they experienced leading and co-leading in triads, what else they learned professionally during the workshop, and what they plan to do to maintain their professional gains. Next, they are asked what they gained personally and what they will do to maintain their personal gains.

A final fantasy trip: "Shut your eyes and imagine you are at home. Remember that small children will tell you how much they missed you by pointing out everything that went wrong in your absence and some partners will do the same. How will you show... not tell... the ways you have changed?

"Be at your office. People may or may not be interested in what you learned. Share with those who are interested."

"Don't burn up on reentry."

Now is the time for personal strokes and sharing.

I make sure there are special strokes for the organizers, all who brought food or fulfilled other tasks, and very special strokes for any translators. Group members stroke me. All of us stand up, hug, and give private strokes. Then, if this is part of the structure, we party together.

THREE

Nature and Nurture*

*Some of this material first appeared in *Redecision Therapy* journal.

In redecision therapy clients reenact childhood scenes in order to effect changes in themselves in the present. In reliving these scenes they make new decisions about themselves, called redecisions. As a framework for therapy, this injunction-decision-redecision model is excellent. Whether the scenes are true, confabulations, or the typical fictionalized memories of early childhood, clients use them to make dramatic and lasting changes in themselves. The theory works. And it is not fact.

When I was learning to be a therapist, everyone blamed mothers for their children's emotional and behavioral problems. When a child was autistic, mothers were told it was their fault and the only hope for the child was psychoanalysis ... of the mother. Homosexuality was caused by domineering ("castrating") mothers. Asthma and stomach aches were caused by over-protective mothers. Schizophrenia was caused by faulty family communication. Although the importance of fathers finally began to be acknowledged by family therapists, therapists still wrote papers on "schizophrenigenic mothers."

Our view of injunctions-decisions is also based on a prejudiced view of families, inasmuch as we have ignored clients' innate characteristics while encouraging the clients to see parents and parental figures as villains who give injunctions and thereby pave the way for the clients' problems in adult life.

I am convinced that within a very few years scientists will have discovered the exact genetic causes of autism and all psychoses. Genetic influences on personality and character structure will also be found. Why has the world of psychotherapy taken so long in acknowledging a fact that every lay person has always known, that each person is intrinsically unique from birth? Have we hung back because we know that clients find therapy more palatable when they can blame their parents rather than their genes?

The transactional analysis thinking was: children are born princes and princesses, and turned into frogs by the witch messages of their parents. Therapists and their clients have been pleased with this idea, just as they are pleased with the concept of the hurting, pathetic, delicate, and infinitely boring *inner child.* Blaming parents continues to be stylish.

In real life it's sometimes the other way around. Some children are born froggie, while quite healthy parents may become psychologically impaired as they try to raise their difficult children.

Everyone knows that each baby is different. One is placid and happy, another merely placid. Some babies are characterized as sad, others as angry. Babies may be restless or irritable, easily frightened, contact-eager or contact-spurning. There are seemingly healthy babies who cry every time they are put down, as well as those who seldom cry. Children and parents have the job of figuring out how to live together, and it may be difficult. The ideal is a family in which everyone is happy, loving, and productive, but that isn't easy. For example, it is difficult for a family of type A adults to appreciate their type B baby. The child is so slow! And what's he got to be so calm about? This is not a family who welcomes a Buddha. A different child, hyperactive and even irritable, would fit in better, but that same child would be devastating to an overwhelmed, tired, or chronically ill single parent. A good fit enhances a child's self-esteem, but also may cement innate character traits that turn out to be undesirable in adult life. Clients' difficulties and unhappiness result from a complicated combination of nurture and nature.

Our theory of Child decisions postulates that each child makes unique decisions in response to injunctions. A decision may be an acceptance of an injunction: Don't be—I'll kill myself; a rejection of an injunction: Don't be close—I am close to many people even if I am not close to you; a partial compliance or rejection: Don't succeed—I'll discount my successes but I'll make more money than you ever could. There are addenda to decisions concerning how the person feels or behaves toward the injunction-giver: I'll hate you forever and blame you whenever anything goes wrong; I'll spend my life trying to make you love me or trying to make you happy. Transactional analysis and redecision theory are useful guides in therapy for therapists who don't make a religion of them.

As therapists we are often amazed at the health and strength of clients who survived terrible trauma in their own homes. It is also noteworthy that some clients, who are quite ill psychologically, were raised in seemingly healthy, nurturing, supportive environments.

Why do children respond so differently? There are a few obvious answers. The child who is beautiful, has a pleasing personality, or is especially intelligent will be more apt to get positive responses than unattractive children. Children with chronically snotty noses tend to be pushed away by all but the most adoring parents. It certainly is nice to be admired in childhood. Children who are intrinsically happy may be predisposed to ignore injunctions. Unhappy children make poorer decisions for themselves and are certainly more fine-tuned to hear injunctions. If they have flunked childhood in some important way, they have to decide to blame themselves or blame others. If they flunk adulthood, the same is true. Either way, they have a harder time liking themselves.

Each child's inherent personality is at least as important in the fashioning of decisions as are the injunctions the child receives. In fact, it might be argued that a child's personality and character structure may become the bearer of injunctions. A genetically depressed child may be both giver and receiver of "Don't exist" messages. Children who don't bond (the autistic child, for example) give "Don't be close" messages to self and to anyone who wants to love them.

Here are examples of two clients whose decisions about themselves may be based on their own inherent character structure.

Don't be happy.

Charles is a bright, good looking, irritable, and very unhappy young adult. He consistently blames others for his problems. His belief is, "If they had only done ____ instead of ____ I would now be happy." His parents gave him many of the things he thought would bring happiness, but he remained as unhappy as ever. When he read *Changing Lives*, he was immediately excited and signed up for a workshop. By the time he arrived, he had collected dozens of scenes that explained his unhappiness and proved that he had been given every injunction in the book by his parents, teachers, and other adults.

As we traced his life stories, we realized he didn't seem to remember ever being happy for more than a few hours at a time. He didn't display symptoms of a serious underlying depression nor could he be labeled paranoid. He was an unhappy man who blamed others for his unhappiness.

During the workshop his therapist said, "You know about diabetes… lack of production or utilization of body insulin. I think you have a similar disease. Don't discount this. It seems safe to say that your happiness quotient is far below normal. Some bio-chemical may be lacking in your brain, so you lack the natural ability to experience happiness. You can get pharmaceuticals to elevate your mood on a permanent basis. Or you can make a contract with yourself to figure out if there is any way you can make yourself happy in spite of this seeming deficit. Want to give it a shot?"

When the patient agreed, more than a bit skeptically, he was told to reenter the early scenes in which he had previously worked. This time, instead of finding the injunctions and fighting against them, he was simply to pretend he was born with a huge supply of happiness genes.

The first scene was the birth of his baby sister. Instead of his previous bitter unhappiness at being pushed out of babyhood too soon, he imagined himself playing with his toys in a very sunny room and scarcely noticing her existence. With a little help from his therapist, he imagined himself happy with his parents and imperturbable with his sister. He was astonished. "I think we've got something here! Because it's true… it's like I was predestined not to be happy." He redid several scenes and began appreciating the quality of happiness, which he named "an alternate life style." He wanted to be happy and worked hard toward that goal, but his happiness was largely intellectual. He didn't experience a natural joy, although he certainly began being nicer to himself and others. He remained a serious young man. He reported that whenever he had a problem in his current life, he would ask himself, "How would a happy man handle this?"

Don't be the sex you are.

In the movie "Mi Vie En Rose" a young boy insists he is a girl, and is a dazzlingly beautiful girl when he dresses the part. A very boyish-looking girl, who also likes to cross-dress, wears his clothes. The movie underlines societal prejudice and the inherent nature of gender identity disorders (defined in the DSM IV as "the desire to be, or the insistence one is, of the other sex.")

If their parents had believed in psychotherapy, the movie children might have been sent to a therapist who was willing to take on the task of curing their sexual identity disorder. Like the offensive neighbors in the movie, such a therapist would be one more person who did not accept the children as they were.

Would the story have been different if this boy had been a large, muscular kid who in no way could look stereotypically feminine? When he looked in the mirror he'd see a homely but tough little boy wearing lipstick. And what if the girl had been a fragile, petite child? How important are stereotyped notions about physical appearance?

Jean came into therapy because of mild but uncomfortable depression and feelings of worthlessness even though she was successful in her marriage and her career. Certainly, she had received and accepted the injunction, "Don't be the sex you are." Her father had taught her to "pitch a baseball like a boy," and they had fished and attended sports events together. He invented a boy's nickname for her and used it exclusively. When he was dying, he told her, "I've always been sorry you're not a man. You are too intelligent to be a woman."

She remembers her absolute belief from about age four, "I am a boy with a girl's body." She was uninterested in girls or in girls' games. She identified with males in real life, books, and movies. Her mother and grandmother attempted to make her "more feminine" by choosing frilly clothes for her and sending her to ballet classes, but her own inner conviction prevailed. Throughout childhood she told herself, "When I grow up I will wear men's clothing and then everybody will think I am a man." When she reached adolescence she gave up her fantasy and became severely depressed.

This seems an obvious example of an injunction and decision, but Jean says it is not. Although she can't define what constitutes a male personality, she knows that she experiences herself as masculine rather than feminine. She is quite certain her masculinity is inborn and that her father, wanting a son, recognized this inborn masculinity.

In therapy she created scenes in which she fought back against stereotypes, insisting she was OK without frills and ballet. She seemed to have found psychological peace. "I am a married woman, a female, and I love the woman I've become. I was a gutsy little girl-boy who grew up to be a fine woman." She was not as satisfied as she thought she was. Later, in a therapy workshop she wonders, "Would I have been happier if my parents had known and accepted my secret belief that I am really male?" She plays out an imaginary scene in which she tells her father her secret, "I am a boy in a girl's body." She is startled as she hears herself say, as her father, "I wanted a real boy, a son. I was disappointed not to have a real son, but you and I had fun together. You were a tomboy." As her mother, Jean says, "I, too, am disappointed. I wanted a real girl, who'd let me curl her hair and dress her up. I do love you just the same."

In a moving, emotional scene Jean responds, "You both say I am not real. I'm not a real boy or a real girl. You are both disappointed in me. I've always known you felt that way. No wonder I felt worthless."

It is suggested that she be a new parent for her child. She agrees, and holds a pillow to represent herself as a child. "I am not disappointed in you. You are real and very precious. I love you, little boy in a girl's body. I love myself, a man in a woman's body."

The question remains.

Are injunctions and decisions real or imaginary?

Are injunctions given only by outsiders or also by the child's unique genetic or biochemical make-up?

No matter how "objective" a client or therapist wants to be, the patient's memories and belief system plus the therapist's belief system will color both theory and therapy. The best therapy occurs when the therapist is willing to listen well and when both therapist and client have the freedom to explore the client's world with as little prejudice as possible.

FOUR

Old Age

I've reached old age. The date was not a matter of age or health. The onset of Old Age is idiosyncratic and in my case nonsensical. There were signposts along the way. Physical and mental trauma. Diminished memory. The deaths of my husband and friends. Tiredness. Aching legs and hips. Loss of all hope for our political system. And lots of little things, like how do you re-set the right-hand margin on the computer?

But none of these defined Old Age for me. Then one day some Mexican guys helped me into the warm, calm, wonderful waters of Isla Mujeres... and I couldn't swim. I could paddle, of course, in a dumb, baby way, but real swimming was gone forever. Never again could I scuba dive, snorkel, take mile-long swims. No real swims at all. I couldn't wear flippers without getting immediate muscle cramps and my legs just fiddled around in the water, getting me nowhere. The guys, always helpful, suggested Doña Mari could use a life vest. I cried inside. Old Age had happened.

It's not the end of my world. Strangely, life continues to be a lot of fun. Much in my old age is still beautiful. First, though, the negative, which began to set in early, while I was still just merely old.

Health

I am in a hospital, brought there by my son and daughter. I am conscious and in a frightened, intolerable turmoil. Through the strangeness of my new world I hear a question, asked by a doctor I don't know "What year is this?" I want to answer and am doing what seems like thinking. Aren't the 1900s over? I think and think and think and I am not sure. I don't want to be wrong, so I say nothing. I feel like a child who cannot answer a teacher's question. I am humiliated. In childhood I always knew the answers, shouted them out, drove teachers batty with my loud knowledge, and now I do not know what year it is. I try to try to remember. "Who is president of the United States?" this doctor continues. "The worst man in the world," I say happily, knowing I got that answer right. But he asks me the president's name. I can't remember. My son intervenes. "Don't ask her these questions. She doesn't even know my name."

I am stricken. I want so much to reassure him that I know his name. He is my son, my first baby. How could I not know his name? I start to cry. If you want an example of terrible shame, it is the realization that you don't know your own son's name.

The next day I wake up feeling fine and insist on leaving the hospital. Afterwards I discover that I can't type because I no longer remember the keyboard. I also can't do crossword puzzles because I have lost or misplaced so many words from my vocabulary. I spend all day every day typing, reading, and doing crossword puzzles, until I am back to normal.

When I was a new MSW, I worked at a county hospital. Every Friday afternoon I was in charge of intake for the emergency psychiatry ward. In my arrogance I asked poor old people the terrible questions, as I was taught to do, "Who is president?" "What year is it?" "What city is this?" "Count backwards by sevens from 100." I didn't consider that my questions shamed them. I didn't realize that their condition, called "not oriented as to time and place," might be temporary. They might have awakened that morning in a turbulent confusion, as I had, or they might have been wandering the streets for months in this condition. These old men and women should have been taken immediately to a medical ward, but they weren't wanted there. Maybe some of them were reacting to extraordinarily high blood pressure and were suffering, as I had, a small, transient stroke. They would respond quickly to medical procedures. Or perhaps they were reacting to medicine they should not have been given. Whatever the cause of their current mental dysfunction, a new social worker should not have been assessing them. They should not have ended up on a psychiatric ward, receiving no treatment, simply because they were poor. There was so much I didn't know then, including that these people who failed the tests might feel the anguish of their predicament but be unable to tell me that. What goes around comes around.

Following one of my hip surgeries, I was sent to a convalescent institution with an inspiring name. If you are a senior, beware of places with names such as A Home For Mom, Autumn Glow, Compassionate Care, Home Sweet Home, Eden Place. Supposedly, I was sent to the best facility in the county for care plus physical therapy. Some of you may be working with clients who live in the worst in the county. I cannot even imagine what such places are like. So here I am in the wing for people like me, who need physical therapy and care. Another part of this facility is for the chronically ill. I know they could use physical therapy, too, but instead they are tied into their wheelchairs each morning and placed in front of television sets they do not watch.

I share a tiny room with a woman who talks all the time, banally, about her various surgeries. I am not paid to be her social worker and my hip hurts too much for me to consider doing volunteer work. She has the bed by the window and I can't see out. The food is not vegetarian and is by my standards inedible. All of it. My grand-daughter comes to visit. "Gramma, what have they done to you? Why are you here? There is a man dying right near your room, and nobody is paying any attention!" Unfortunately for him, he is not dying. He is one of the chronics, who may sit there for years with his tongue hanging out. "You can't stay here!" I agree.

She gives me her cell phone and I leave a message with my surgeon that I will not spend one more hour in this place. I tell him I am leaving for the day with my grand-daughter and will return to check out permanently before bedtime. If he and they don't discharge me, I will simply be AWOL. I do know that going AWOL means Medicare will punish both the doctor and me.

When I return in the evening, the discharge papers are ready for me. I move into my daughter's home and a physical therapist sees me there. Compared to many old people, I am very lucky. I have a wonderful granddaughter and a daughter who will take me in. Also, I am stubborn.

You know you are old when you walk very slowly and are desperately afraid of falling. Both of my hips have broken and been replaced. The arteries in my legs are clogged as a result of long term diabetes. People tell me, as they hold a door open, "Take your time. Don't hurry." I am the epitome of a Type A personality encased in a

Type D-minus body. If I could, I would love to hurry. I dream of running. But I keep my eyes on the sidewalk in front of me and remain afraid.

Since then, I have had two bad falls, both times had to return to the use of a walker and, if it weren't for the laser-puncture and other treatment I receive in Cuba twice a year, I would not be walking much at all. I lost the sight in my right eye temporarily from the wet type of macular degeneration, but recently they have found a successful treatment for this curse. I see fairly well. I don't hear well. From this moment until the day I die, I know it's a downhill trip.

Finances

I have lost my money through a stupid investment. I do worry. I wrote a book that sold quite well, called *Not To Worry*, so consider myself an expert on the subject. I know all the antidotes for worry and practice them one at a time. I don't feel humiliated by my financial failures; in fact, being a socialist, I used to feel humiliated at having money. I am not as concerned now as many people think I should be. I scheduled final workshops in Mexico and Arizona this year (2007), which brought in cash. Some wonderful friends are making it possible for me to take another trip to Cuba.

In 1944 when I was nineteen I moved alone to Mexico City. My father mailed me my money, which I had earned as a waitress on the steamship North America, because he believed this was safer than my carrying it on my person. He was wrong. It didn't arrive for several months. Long before that, I gave my last ten centavos to a beggar, because that amount was truly worthless even then, and persuaded the people with whom I lived to let me stay until my money arrived, which was very kind of them considering that we didn't know each other well and they were poor. Without bus fare I walked miles to classes. The only bothersome problem was that I could not buy wood to heat water for a shower. During this period, I wasn't the least bit worried. Like everything else I experienced during my six months in Mexico, it was part of the adventure. Today, although I do worry, I find my financial problem mildly adventurous.

For many people lack of money is a nightmare. I remember this from my job at the county. I would phone welfare, talk with my client's worker, with the worker's supervisor, the supervisor's supervisor, people I knew from Democratic politics. It could take hours to get a rule modified so that a client and her family would be guaranteed enough to eat... for a while anyway. My clients truly could not do this for themselves. Their nightmare was constant. The problems of poverty take precedent over all others except emergency medical care. The two may go hand in hand.

As with poor health, I maintain a somewhat humorous attitude toward my lack of money. It's bad enough to be hurting and poor, without also being depressed or angry.

Housing

Because of the loss of my savings, I have given up my beautiful apartment that faces San Francisco Bay. I probably can no longer afford to live anywhere in San Francisco. I've lost my favorite city, where buses and taxis take one anywhere, the only place in the world where I have wanted to live permanently. Truth is, I left it several years ago simply to travel the world, but now that walking is difficult, traveling forever seems impossible. So I moved back, the rent increased mightily, and now again I have left. My furniture, paintings, and books are in my daughter's home in Oregon, so I can visit and feel at home. I am living with a friend in Berkeley, just a short rapid transit ride to San Francisco. I love it here.

Some friends and family believe I should enter an assisted living arrangement because of my age, my eyes, my hips, and the fact that I might fall again. One of Bob's and my partners from Western Institute days recently told me of an assisted living arrangement that I would like. His mother-in-law likes it. I know her to be the compliant type. I told him I would rather be dead. My grandson John says his other grandmother is in a place I would like. He described the beautiful new furniture. I explained, "If I am to go to jail, I want to go to a real jail, even though the furniture is not new. In a real jail there are people who are still fighting and still interesting. I will not live in a pseudo jail that is fancied up nicely so that people won't notice that the front doors are locked."

A variety of people want to think for me. I fought hard against being treated as a child when I was a child. Imagine me letting someone treat me as a child today! There are worse things than fighting fate. Anyway, I can't afford assisted living, fortunately. A friend has just given me enough money to see me through this year. She insists I tell no one. How do you sufficiently thank a person for such incredible generosity?

Other Losses

Bob Goulding has been dead fourteen years. For a long time, his death blotted out anything good in life. Now I am used to living without him. I remember him with love and relive in memory romantic and funny times together. I talk to others about his abilities as a therapist.

All of us old ones have had major losses. Too many friends and colleagues are physically incapacitated, senile, or dead. Parents, grandparents, uncles, and aunts are long dead, of course. It's strange how often they, like Bob, are in my dreams. I am an atheist, but take comfort in the knowledge that memories live and can be passed down to the younger family members. I have my father's stories of his childhood in the early 1900s, my grandfather's stories beginning with the end of the Civil War, and my own stories that are ancient history to my grandchildren.

I am lucky that all four of my sisters survive, though three brothers-in-law have died. My son and daughters get older every year, which amazes me. I expect everyone else to age, but not my ex-children. They are good friends now. Even my grandchildren are adults. There are nieces and nephews who might have been lost to me if it were not for the miracle of e-mail. Transactional Analysis friends are also accessible with the click of the e-mail. I send and receive messages from all over the United States, from Sweden, Mexico, Cuba, Japan, Ireland, Canada, Australia, and Peru. This is the richness of belonging to an international organization.

And speaking of being blessed, I have a very special, secret love of my own. So far old age is at worst tolerable and sometimes it's truly wonderful... even though I can no longer swim worth a damn.

FIVE

Some Injunctions of Old Age

Don't Be Close

Some therapists don't retire because their major closeness is to their patients. Alan Wheelis, psychoanalyst, wrote, "For some people the problem of intimacy is the principle determinant of the vocational choice of psychoanalysis. The conflict is between the tendencies that lead to closeness and the fear that is evoked by closeness." He went on, "Lean hands within him reach out hungrily. He longs to touch, to feel, to warm himself by this bright fire, so close, so near, so unutterably far away. Though perhaps always slightly out of reach for themselves, psychoanalysts believe love and closeness is achievable. And to some extent they lessen the man-made misery of man. Hatred they endure and do not turn away. Love comes their way and they are not seduced. They are the listeners, and their silence is not cold." To me this statement is unbearably sad.

When a child loses a parent, the child may decide, "I'll never be close to anyone again because it hurts too much when they leave." A lifetime of emotional distance may ensue.

Early injunctions and decisions do not account for most of the loneliness of old age. The "Don't be close" messages in old age come from recent losses. The longer a person lives, the more family members and friends are gone from their lives. People experience what feels like an onslaught of desertions without the psychological strength to start over.

Therapy: Treat the depression first. Group therapy is of great value and small group meetings should be a part of every assisted living facility. Old people need something to do and people to talk with. Encourage intimate relationships, sexual and psychological. Intimacy enhances life for the very old, as it does for everyone. If a sexual relationship is not possible, let your clients know that masturbation is health-enhancing.

There may be multiple good-byes to be experienced in therapy. A good-bye can be imagined at the place of their last meeting, the funeral parlor, or the graveside. Let the client take the time necessary. Resentments and appreciations are given, and client ends with the words "you are dead" or "you are no longer in my life."

Don't Want

People who have accepted this injunction have a hard time asking for help. They don't complain. Being sweet may leave them at the end of the line when goodies or even essential health services are being delivered. They are proud of not asking for wheelchairs at airports, cheap taxi coupons, or handicapped parking.

Therapy: Help your clients to know what they want or need, to ask for what they want, and then to accept the help they are given. They may need to learn whom to ask for what, and when to compromise. Therapy will almost always include learning to give to themselves.

Don't Be A Child

Their role was to be little parents to their infantile real parents or to their younger siblings. Retired, they may enjoy being in the ranks of the volunteers, finding unpaid jobs in which they can still take care of others. This may be a good way to spend retirement years, but people are often frustrated when their attempts to help are not sufficiently appreciated, or when they grow too old or too incapacitated to be care-givers. Even at this late date, they may have a vague hunch that there is more to life than parenting.

Therapy: Don't try to change your client. The world needs givers! However, you and your client may want to explore additional options for living life richly and happily. A pleasant goal during therapy is to laugh together or, better yet, giggle during each session. As your clients become incapacitated, they'll need to realize that it is sometimes more important to receive than to give.

Don't Have Fun

As children, some people worked constantly, got good grades, and then became doctors or executives who never took time off. Unlike the rest of their colleagues, they didn't use their money for fancy vacations and better toys. Their work was their life. When their work ends, they may wander back to their place of employment to prove to themselves (if not to those still working) that they are still needed. They don't recognize the pleasure in going to the movies in the middle of the day, walking in a lovely park, or doing nothing at all. They ask tensely, "But what shall I do with the rest of my life?" Sometimes they find a hobby, like golf or politics, which they can pursue full time with the same drive they showed in their working years.

Therapy: Of course it's OK to help such clients find volunteer work, second careers, golf instructors, or personal trainers to help them structure their time. Perhaps they would also like to write their memoirs or family history. I help them get in touch with their internal and infernal Parental voices, which probably are still telling them to work hard. They can have an interesting, personally valuable time playing with and zonking these Critical Parent voices. Redecision therapy works well. These elders, who have always been successful, can be superb, successful clients. Make sure they practice their new found freedom to make friends and establish intimate bonds

There is another group of people who neither have fun nor have experienced success. If you have worked with them when they were children and adolescents, you will recognize them when they are wrinkled. They have always found the shit rather than the pony.

Therapy: They are usually lonely and often have been lonely for years. Contact with a therapist is itself therapeutic, even though they probably complain at therapy's ineffectiveness. Perhaps you can help them laugh during therapy, at least once in a while. Look for ways to give these clients positive strokes and teach them to accept your strokes. If you have a good, strong group, bring them into it. The group will offer them an opportunity to experience the art of socialization and the art of having fun. (Read the chapter "Nature and Nurture" and perhaps help your client "work hard" at being happy.)

Do not pin a "don't have fun" label on those whose major problem is pain. Suffering cancels out fun in anyone's life. Hurting clients need pain relief before anything else.

Don't Be Old

This injunction is given by advertisements for cosmetics, anti-wrinkle creams, by countless books and magazine articles espousing health, exercise, and nutrition. Beauticians, plastic surgeons, nutritionists, and personal trainers all advertise that they can help you regain or maintain your "youth" even though you are some sixty years beyond the definition of "young." Friends and family say "Don't be old" when they insist that you haven't changed a bit or that you look younger than ever!

When people tell me "You don't look *that* old." I say, "I am eighty-two. This is how eighty-two looks on me." It is more relaxing to be the age I am than to try to be an age I am not. On the other hand, I knew a woman who had her final face lift at ninety-three and she did look great. Many men and women dye their hair forever. That is fine. So is tossing out the make-up, dye, and plastic surgery appointments.

Therapy: Therapy certainly won't make a client young, so what else is new? Go for the contract a person chooses, and don't get hung up with issues of age unless age is used as an excuse for not having a good life. Then the first contract becomes a "contract of exploration." What might the client do, think, believe, feel that would enhance life in spite of old age? Clients may use childhood scenes, when grandparents were aged, to make redecisions for themselves today.

Don't Be Important

We are supposed to be wise and yet our opinions are discounted. Much of what we know is obsolete. Some people prattle on about the wisdom of age, but they don't really mean it. (And if you examine our Congress people and Supreme Court judges, you will notice that nobody gets wiser as they age. The stupid remain stupid beyond belief.) It is difficult to feel important when family and friends ignore your ideas, while trying to impose on you their own ideas of what you should or could be doing, or if they simply treat you like a piece of furniture to be moved and cleaned periodically.

Therapy: From the first "hello" the therapist will listen and work with the person to form a therapy contract. This in itself is an invaluable message that the client is important. When the client decides to assert her or his importance, it is best to practice it first with the therapist. People who are unused to asserting their own importance may use self-negating words or body language, and may give up too easily. Another goal is to learn self-esteem.

Don't Be

I assume Ernest Hemingway suffered from an intractable depression that had genetic components. Others in his family have also committed suicide. A hard drinker, he stayed vigorously alive through his early and middle adult years. His final depression may have been a reaction to his inability to reconcile himself to old age. We can guess that his internal programming was, "Be a real man," which means "be successful, strong, heroic, play and drink hard, and write the world's best books." I am guessing his depression overwhelmed him when he could no longer live up to his "real man" definitions.

Old age is not easy. Depression is just around each corner, beckoning. The desire to die may result from loneliness, depression, trauma, pain, losses, and incapacitation. There are alternatives to suicide. Loneliness is not a reason for dying, but is a reason for learning new ways to make friends. Whatever the age, depression is treatable. Pain medications are more effective than they used to be. Hospice is a choice that allows living with dignity and achieving a meaningful farewell to the living before a relatively peaceful death.

Sometimes, in spite of all help that is available, an individual is simply tired of living and ready to die. My father reached that point when he could no longer hold a book. He'd gone from serious literature to the OZ books he knew from childhood. He looked at picture books.

He invented his very own Walter Mitty stories with himself as hero. Now he was done. Fortunately, he had a compassionate and prejudice-free doctor who let him die of pneumonia, assisted by morphine to offset discomfort.

Therapy: Therapists who are willing to listen without prejudice can be truly helpful to elderly clients facing a choice of living or dying.

References:

Allen B. Wheelis, *Quest for Identity*, W.W. Norton, 1959.

SIX

What are You Doing with the Rest of Your Life?*

*Some of this material first appeared in *Redecision Therapy* journal.

What are our choices in retirement years? To retire? To keep on working? To semi-retire? To redirect? It's a blank page and yet not always blank. Sometimes old instructions shine through, like the palimpsest in which Archimedes' words are still legible behind prayers written in the Middle Ages. In our choices today we can sometimes read the choices of our ancestors. I decided to ask friends and colleagues what they learned about retirement and being old from observing their grandparents and other relatives when they were children. And how does what they learned then affect them now? Here are some answers given by psychotherapist friends.

My grandfather was forced to retire from the military at age 65. He was a dentist. I have a collection of his letters, including those in which he begged the Army to reinstate him. He didn't care about the money. He wanted to be useful. He died in his late 80's while helping my father edit a book. His slogan was, "As long as you're needed, you won't die." In my late 80's I am still writing and editing a book.

My grandfather decided to retire when I was a baby. He told his four sons that they would have to support him. My father was the eldest, but he was not wealthy so it was very hard on him. My grandfather had a fine time, inviting his friends to tea and chatting with them, but my mother had to sell her jewelry to support his life style. I decided that when I grew up no one was ever going to have to support me!

My father worked as long as he could, because he loved his work and his work was admired all over the country. When he retired he became massively depressed. He was hospitalized and given shock treatment, but he never fully recovered. I have not considered retiring.

My mother was like an aging actress. She lived for applause and adulation. She never had a profession, but was president of this organization or that. She used to introduce famous writers who came to town to speak or spoke herself for local charities. But as she became old and crippled from arthritis, where could she find applause? She became depressed and nothing seemed to help. There is a huge difference between being liked and being applauded. She was liked, but needed applause. To tell you the truth, I am just like her. I went back into therapy at age seventy to learn how to give myself enough applause to keep going.

My grandfather had a bad heart. After his heart attack, he took good care of himself for awhile, letting the young men at the store do the heavy work. He didn't want to be called a shirker so gradually he began working as hard as the others, and died of his second heart attack. It's damned if you do, damned if you don't, my family says. That may be why I have so much trouble making decisions about retirement.

In our family poverty threatened our very existence. There was no social security, no Medicare, and anything you saved might be stripped away in a moment. The only asset we had was the ability to work. As I think about it, I realize I am behaving as if that were true for me, even though I have more money than I can possibly spend in my lifetime.

My father faked a back injury to retire from the police force before he was fifty. My grandfather said, "He ought to pull his own weight." I was disgusted with my father. I don't plan to retire, so I do what my grandfather did, keep working while being contemptuous of my lazy, happy colleagues.

My father was a business executive. He had to be boss. When he retired, they moved to a retirement community. Instead of having an easy life, he spent his time organizing everything there, bossing people around, forming committees and more committees. He was tireless! When others finally pushed him out and took over, he went to bed and chose to die. I was always a failure in his eyes, so I had the freedom to choose a happy life before and after retirement. I taught school, traveled, and had fun with my family. When people asked me if I thought I would be bored when I retired, I reminded them, "I've practiced retirement every summer for thirty years, so by now I should be pretty good at it."

When father retired, mother couldn't stand having him around the house all day. He sat in the kitchen if she was in the kitchen and followed her all over the house. He sat and watched mother and her friends play bridge. Neither was happy.

My grandmother said, "I would be ashamed to go to Florida and do nothing but play bridge." She was a Calvinist, so doing anything enjoyable smacked of sinfulness. I don't want to be like her, but it's an uphill battle. I work like hell at not being useful!

My father's brother retired at 55. He had a fine life, playing golf and just having a good time. He was the only person in the family who laughed a lot. My father considered him a bum. I chose to be like my uncle. I retired as soon as possible and major in Elderhostel. Like my uncle, I have a great time.

When my mother died, my father retired and spent his life traveling. I resented that my mother missed out on the good times and vowed I would not be cheated by death. I asked myself what I wanted from life and I am already giving it to myself.

My grandfather told us that the saddest thing in life was to die before you had time to enjoy retirement.

I think of my family as a river that flows forever. All men and most women work outside the home. Mothers or grandmothers may stay home to take care of the children. Women retire when they are needed to take care of the old ones. The unmarried women may work outside the home a few years longer than the rest, but they also retire to be caretakers. Some in our family need perpetual care, like my nephew who is retarded. There really isn't such a thing as actual retirement, because we start life being cared for, work at home or at a job, take care of others, and then end up being taken care of. Along the way there are celebrations and reunions and many happy times. Sometimes one of us goes off for a spell. When we take a vacation to one of the national parks or to Europe, we bring back postcards and souvenirs for those who prefer to stay home.

I asked my grandmother, who had a terrible marriage, how it was to be old and alone. I must have been about ten at the time. She said, "It is better than heaven. I am free and I don't have to take care of anyone. Just pray you make it, honey. Old age is the best time of all." She stayed happy the rest of her life. I now relish my freedom and lack of responsibilities.

The grown-ups in my family work in order to save for their retirements, just as we children ate our meat and vegetables in order to have dessert. Retirement is the dessert of life.

In my family lots of people get second jobs after they retire. My father worked in a bank, because my grandfather owned the bank, and then the bank was bought out and my father became a specialist in buying and selling antique furniture. My aunt retired from nursing and began writing romances. My mother joined the library board so that she could read every book and decide which ones the library should buy. I am only sixty-five and I've already been a probation officer, an English teacher, a psychotherapist, and now I play around with computers.

I talked with others who either didn't know or care about directives from the past. They are simply doing what they do.

The joy of semi-retirement is that I no longer need to deal with managed care. Managed care requires that a therapist publicly damn her clients with diagnoses that will cling to them for the rest of their lives. That is what I retired from. I take reduced fees in cash only. I feel very sorry for young therapists who never knew therapy without managed care.

After retirement, I redirected my life. I have always loved art, so I got a master's degree in art and am now a docent at the Museum of Modern Art. I also take one art tour a year.

I manage on a welfare budget, because I lost all my assets when I became crippled and legally blind before I was eligible for Medicare. I studied the system and am proud of how well I use it. I wangled from Social Services one of the few adequate welfare apartments in a safe area. That is no mean feat in San Francisco. I have Meals on Wheels plus daily housekeeper service. I fought successfully for an electric wheel chair so I can scoot happily around my neighborhood. I receive reduced-fee taxi service, which I use for trips to the hospital and to attend free university courses. I am often given two free tickets to operas and concerts, and give the second ticket to anyone willing to drive me there. I sign up for every free cultural experience I can find. I get free audio books for the blind, and really enjoy them. You could say that I have a terrible life, but I am making the best of it.

I quit my job, bought a trailer, and now travel around the country building houses for Habitat for Humanity. I got tired of intellectual work and I am a good carpenter. Physical work keeps me healthy.

Where can a retired elder live independently, with lively company of all ages, and get help when it is needed? Let me tell you about the place I have chosen. It is an old-fashioned type village with some new features that make it a caring, peaceful community. We planned the buildings and layout: cars on the perimeter, gardens and flowered walkways between houses, community vegetable garden, pool. The clubhouse has guest rooms, a children's' play room, teen room, lounge, music room, dining room, and kitchen. The land on the surrounding acreage is left wild.

All decisions were and are made by consensus so agreement is guaranteed. (One can vote "yes" and mean I hate that idea but, as it is important for you, I will not block it.) Does it take a lot of time to make community decisions? Sure it does. Is it worth it? Yes.

We eat in our own homes or in the clubhouse ($2 to $4 a meal). We play billiards, ping pong, scrabble, run, attend onsite movies, and play music with friends. You dream it up and it can happen here.

I used to stew about retirement while not retiring. Luckily for me, retirement was forced on me by company rules. After I stopped working, I discovered all the things I wanted to do. Coffee with friends, hiking, reading, playing chess. I take Greyhound to explore parts of the country I'd never seen. I have a fine life.

I am seventy-two and am finding this business of getting old rather interesting. Now that I look old and safe, lots of women smile at me. Waitresses call me "Hon." Yes, I am still working full time and enjoying it. A whole new world has opened for me, the world of dancing. When I was six, I explained to my parents that I was never going back to church because the music was terrible. Lately, I tried aerobics but the exercises are boring and the music as bad as the church music of my childhood. I like dance music and the exercise of dancing. Also, amazingly, I am very good at it. I am silver level in American Ballroom and go to Buenos Aires to study tango dancing. I love Buenos Aires. Nobody cares that my Spanish is terrible so long as I can tango well.

This is difficult to explain, but my life is becoming more coherent and congruent. I am making my own version of my life and I like this version. Included in the new version is a mystical vision I experienced when I was with a group of Coptic Christians, touring Turkey.

My wife is dead, and yet we still have a relationship. For me it is a peaceful awareness of her absence which, though I cannot explain it, seems to keep us close.

I noticed I was muttering angrily under my breath as I cooked dinner after coming home from work. Curious, because I like to cook. Then I realized that this was one more task I had taken over from my partner, one more task he could no longer physically do. I long for the easy conversations we used to have. His hearing is too impaired to catch the casual quip. Interaction requires forethought on my part. Where had spontaneity gone? I know I can do better than be angry and resentful. After all, I was a therapist who helped others solve similar problems. The next morning, I found for myself a therapist smart enough to say to me all the things I would have said to a patient of mine, and clever enough to laugh with me as she said them. The facts don't change, but it helps me to have someone who will listen to me yell, scream, cry, and laugh about these facts. Anger and resentment make a bad situation worse. That's how it is for me today.

I'm still a happy camper. At seventy-three I sold everything and headed south for a new life in a new country. I live in a house on the beach in Ambergris Caye, Belize. I have all new friends and a new lifestyle. I travel by ferry into town for supplies and by bike to work as a consultant for the Belizean staff at the new grammar school for island kids who otherwise would have no school.

Aging isn't fun, especially when my back pain kicks in, but cheap meds are available as well as plenty of vegetables and fresh fruit... mangos, papayas, avocados, plantains, and coconuts. The negative is not being with my ten-year-old granddaughter (which may be a positive to her parents.) For my seventy-sixth, I flew with friends to Punta Gorda near the Honduras border for a local chocolate festival. A hoot!

Being a caretaker for my wife of sixty years is a mixed blessing. While I cry with deep pain at her changes, I am connected to her in different and profound ways. Seeing that she gets her medicines and vitamins throughout the day, helping her to cook meals, learning to bake with her, and generally keeping house provides for a different kind of closeness.

Although she may ask me ten times a day, "What day is it?", she can drive under my direction, play a mean game of pinochle, and even at times co-lead some of our couples therapy sessions. My wife is always *there* in the present, on top of the subject. Except for when she cried on realizing how much of her memory is gone (during an extensive neurological examination), she is hardly ever unhappy.

I am apprehensive when she is not with me. In new surroundings we stick together like glue. We touch physically more frequently, have very emotionally laden sex, and tell each other how much we love each other very often. It is fulfilling for me when I can turn one of her forgetting moments into a joke and we both laugh. It is also reassuring when I can help her regain her confidence (and memory) in how to ride a bike, play the piano, use a certain kitchen utensil, and care for our plants. I have to weigh how much I should do for her against how much might be infantilizing.

Our coupling style has changed. While there are fewer activities where we function solo, our intimacy is clearly more profound.

SEVEN

I Am Interrupting This Program...*

*Written for the ITAA/USATAA/RTA Conference, 2007

When I was a child listening to the radio, I would occasionally hear the words, "We interrupt this program for an important announcement." This was how I learned that the infamous bank robber Ma Barker was shot dead by Gmen (now called FBI); that the zeppelin Hindenberg had caught fire and crashed... the announcer sobbed, "Oh the humanity, the humanity" and we sobbed with him; that the Lindbergh baby was kidnapped from his bed in the middle of the night; that the Lindbergh baby was returned dead. This is how I learned of Pearl Harbor, the war news, and the death of Roosevelt.

And now I am interrupting this conference program for an important announcement. I am not interrupting to give you updates on today's murders, tortures, oppressions, or other daily horrors that make up our international news. Instead, I am interrupting to give you a way to understand our own part in the problems we face. Ego state pathology explains what makes our daily horrors possible: the combination of prejudiced Parent and evil (or what Eric Berne called fascist) Child, the acceptance of prejudice and evil by the compliant Child, and the advocacy of selfishness instead of altruism by the Child who is naturally selfish and also programmed to be more and more selfish.

The Selfish Child

During the millions of years that human beings were evolving bit by bit over time, I imagine that selfishness was a constant, unchanging necessity. Faced with meager and erratic food supplies and environmental dangers, lacking effective tools, humans needed a combination of cleverness, luck, strength, and especially selfishness for survival. Selfishness, the preoccupation with saving oneself and one's offspring even at the expense of others, would have been essential.

Each of us is a link in a human chain extending back more than five million years. We may know something about our individual great and great-great grandparents, and, if we care, we can trace our ancestry back a few more generations. But five million years! The statistical chance of any one of us having been born is what? Just a trace above zero? Each of us has thousands of direct ancestors and all we know about them is that they lived at least long enough to reproduce.

Shut your eyes and let yourself imagine that you are looking back through time, seeing more and more deeply into your ancestral past. Clothing, languages, tools, facial features, body posture, ways of walking all change. And now you are standing in Africa beside your earliest human ancestors. What a hard time they have surviving. Imagine that miraculously you can communicate with them. You may want to tell them how much we moderns have improved life… in art, literature, varieties of food, tools. We can make cold become hot and hot become cold. We can do so much more to make life easier and richer than they could ever have imagined. And yet… are you embarrassed to tell them that we still behave selfishly even though it is no longer necessary for survival? That so many of our tools are designed solely to annihilate other human beings? How did we ever descend to this?

Back to today. You know the joke about the two hikers who see a bear approaching. One hurriedly takes off his hiking boots and puts on his running shoes. The other says, "You can't outrun a bear." The runner replies, "I only have to outrun you." I detest the gallows humor in that joke. It suggests that we are hard-wired to be selfish rather than altruistic. Although our ancestor's selfishness is no longer necessary, we have not evolved beyond it.

We make some forays into altruism, spending some money on food for the hungry, giving a few street people meager housing, caring for some unfortunate children here and there. Christians have a 2,000-year admonition to love their neighbors as themselves, which is altruism. Few are inclined in this direction, if "neighbor" includes all humans on the planet. Selfishness is ingrown, and we are brainwashed by media injunctions to "Buy More!" From the first moment a child watches television that child is taught to want more and more things. We spend more than we earn, the more the better … on ourselves. We are not altruistic. Our spending is destroying the world and leaving most of the world's people hungry.

The Evil Child

Eric Berne wrote in *What Do You Say After You Say Hello?*:

> "Every human being seems to have a small fascist in his head. This is derived from the deepest layers of the personality (Child in the Child). In civilized people it is usually buried beneath a platform of social ideals and training, but with the proper permissions and directives, as history has shown again and again, it can be liberated into full bloom.... The small fascist is a torturer who probes for and enjoys the weakness of the victim.... It may be said that whoever is not aware of this force in his personality has lost control of it. He has lost control of himself and cannot know where he is headed."

Philip Zimbardo wrote in *The Lucifer Effect*: "Maybe each of us has the capacity to be a saint or sinner, altruistic or selfish, gentle or cruel, dominant or submissive, perpetrator or victim, prisoner or guard." Zimbardo is the professor of social psychology who orchestrated the Stanford University study in the 70s, in which volunteers were randomly selected to be guards or prisoners. The study was scheduled to run for two weeks, but was called off after three days because of the escalating cruelty of the volunteer guards and the psychological deterioration of the volunteer prisoners.

In a later study run by Zimbardo of several dozen "violence workers" (torturers and members of death squads) in Brazil, he found that "these violence workers were ordinary people, not sadists or psychopaths. They were willing to do their jobs because of the training they were given, their group camaraderie, acceptance of the national security ideology, and their learned belief that socialists and communists were enemies of the state." These beliefs about enemies of the state are prejudiced Parent beliefs that support the Evil Child who "committed the most heinous acts under the sanction of the Brazilian government and supported by the CIA."

Let's test ourselves. Imagine that you and I are guards in a prison here or in Iraq. Imagine the odors, the degradation of the prisoners' cloth-

ing compared to ours, the influence on us of the attitudes and actions of other guards, the rules or lack of rules that leave the prisoners at our mercy, the influence of Parental prejudice that says prisoners are criminals or terrorists who deserve punishment. Imagine little by little falling into a pattern of being irritated, arrogant, then angry as we show the prisoners that we are in charge. Imagine committing minor cruelties, then allowing our cruelties to escalate.

As Bob Dylan sang (in the song "George Jackson"):

> "Sometimes I think the whole world
> Is one big prison yard.
> Some of us are prisoners
> The rest of us are guards."

The Compliant Child

If, as Berne suggests, our capacity for cruelty is kept in check by our social idealism and decency, we may believe that we would never humiliate, torture, or kill. Instead, we take the nice road. We are merely observers. Or we back away and pretend not to notice what is going on, what the Evil Child in others is doing. That way, we quietly sanction evil without the shame of committing evil. Think about it. When we don't speak up, we sanction evil ... in our California prisons, in our police forces, in Afghanistan and Iraq and Guatanamo. We do not murder or torture. We stay silent when victims are labeled "collateral damage," "criminals," or "terrorists."

Miguel de Unamuno, the great Spanish philosopher and poet, had the courage to address the Fascists at one of their huge victory celebrations during the Spanish Civil War. He took a microphone and said to them, "At times, to be silent is to lie. You may win because you have enough brute force. But you will not convince. To convince you need to persuade. And in order to persuade you need what you lack: reason and right."

The compliant Adapted Child learns from earliest childhood to obey parents, then teachers, presidents, religious leaders, and everyone else in authority. The Adapted Child obeys in order to be safe and to be loved. "They know what is best for me," the compliant Child often says. Or, "There is nothing I can do... I'm only one person." This part of the personality keeps us quiet observers, afraid even to know that Unamuno was right.

The Prejudiced Parent

The Prejudiced Parent differs from the Critical Parent that all therapists are accustomed to working with. The Critical Parent is an incorporation of the actual parents, older sibs, or teachers. It criticizes self and others; "Your shoes are dirty," "You are so dumb," "Why don't you think before you speak," and is easily defused in therapy.

The Prejudiced Parent is more insidious. I began writing this paper while I was in Cuba with my friend Juan. We were mourning the fact that he will never be able to get a visa to enter the United States even for a brief visit. He asked me, "What would Americans hate most about me? That I'm Cuban? That I'm an atheist? That I'm a communist? Or that I'm Black?"

I said, "The haters would hate you for all those reasons. And you forgot one. You are also poor." As a potential victim of Parental prejudice, he only lacks being Jewish, Moslem, Gay, or female.

Parental prejudice is transmitted by culture and society as well as by actual parents. Hate speeches by political and religious leaders, slanted news in the press and on television, hate blogs, conversations between friends, all may contain Parental prejudice. I was very young when I first read that Jews were tortured to death during the Inquisition. The torture was spelled out in the book I was reading, and I was sick with the horror of it. Later, when studying the Middle Ages, I learned that whole families were put on wooden platforms and burned alive by Catholics who believed that Jews caused epidemics and that Jews drank the blood of Catholic babies. I didn't want to know that people could be so barbarous. (This is the type of horror I never forgot. I had a propensity for imagining myself as one of society's specific victims and suffered quite a lot from this.) It was several years later that all of us found out about the Holocaust.

The Evil Child burned people alive and the Prejudiced Parent told them which people to burn. Without this prejudice against Jews, a poison spread throughout the Christian world, the evil Child in Hitler and his followers could not have carried out the Holocaust. (I liked to think of this as a purely European phenomenon, but our great Franklin Roosevelt turned back the last ship carrying Jews from Europe. The ship was forced to return to Europe, where the people were later rounded up and taken to death camps. Prejudice in the Western Hemisphere caused Eric Berne, among others, to change his name to make it less obviously Jewish. Does anyone not know that his birth name was Bernstein?)

The Poor.

We don't murder the poor and we have outgrown debtors' prisons, but our Parental prejudice and Child selfishness keep them suffering. "It's the poor people's own fault that they are poor. They don't try hard enough," we say. "They don't really want to succeed." "There are rich people who started out poor, so those who remain poor in this land of opportunity are failures, basically inferior people." There is so much anti-poor bias in capitalism that the poor have grown to hate and blame themselves. Did you know that we pay people less for caring for foster children than we pay for boarding horses? As you and I walk on Market Street, San Francisco, threading our way between the homeless, we mostly don't look at them, right? We wish they would go away. We believe that they don't really want homes and warmth and decent clothing.

Atheists.

I often chat with San Francisco taxi drivers, many of whom are Moslems from India or Pakistan. They tell me the good aspects of their religion and assure me that they, too, hate violence. When they get around to talking of the need for tolerance, I agree and mention that I am an atheist. Their tolerance does not extend to atheists. Nor does the tolerance of Christians, I have noticed. Gays and lesbians are elected to public office, but is there a politician anywhere in the US who dares affirm his atheism? I feel a bit let down whenever a candidate announces his candidacy and immediately begins to attend church regularly. I wish just once a politician would say, "I am your best, most qualified candidate, and I do not believe in God." But I know that would be political suicide.

Homosexuals.

When I was in graduate school, gays were still being arrested and sent to "hospitals for the criminally insane," where they were wired up and given electric shock to their genitals. This is called aversion therapy and was advocated by some psychotherapists. Other psychotherapists, including my professors, simply stayed silent about this treatment, just as we stay silent about today's barbarities. Life may be easier for gays, lesbians, and transsexuals than it was fifty years ago, but they are still subject to hate crimes. Self-styled "good people" don't want them to be allowed to marry, join certain churches, or even enter the military. I think this is the only group that remains legally discriminated against.

Race.

I can't imagine that anyone doubts the existence of racial prejudice. If you doubt that you are prejudiced, ask yourself how many of your best friends are of a different race. Do they stop by your home just to say hello? Do you drop by their homes? When race is coupled with poverty, think Katrina. My friend Juan is a retired professional man, soft spoken and gentle. When he heard about Katrina, he seethed with rage. "We are garbage to your government," he said.

Socialism and Communism.

Now let's look at attitudes toward socialism and communism. Anti-Communist propaganda began as soon as the Russian revolution succeeded. Yet, when I was young, communists still paraded proudly in our major cities on Labor Day, although they weren't liked all that much. Our school library had a shelf of socialist and communist literature, and we studied Carl Marx in my eighth grade social studies class.

During the cold war it suddenly wasn't safe even to own Marxist literature. We suffered through McCarthyism, loyalty oaths, public humiliation and loss of work for those accused of being communists.

Politicians ranted against "godless communism," thereby rolling two prejudices into one. Prejudice escalated, aided by the fact that the governments of both the USSR and China were as terrible as governments can be. Unfortunately, no one distinguished between criminal governments and economic theories when thinking about communism. (They did and do distinguish between criminal capitalist governments and capitalism.)

Three and half million people died in the Vietnam War, which we waged to protect us from a peasant communist population that could not possibly have threatened us. In the name of anti-communism, we destroyed decent governments in Guatemala, Iran, Chile, and Nicaragua.

Bush continues to tell Florida Cubans that he plans to invade Cuba to free Cuba from communism and give it democracy. These speeches are on TV and in newspapers in Cuba.

I will tell you about Cuba as I know it. I have been giving workshops in Cuba since January 2002, so I know many therapists in Habana, as well as teachers, translators, and others. It is a poor country with equal but very, very low wages. Cuban communism is based on altruism. What does that mean specifically?

It means that healthcare and education are top notch and free. The percentage of infant, child, and maternal mortality in Cuba is lower than ours. Cuban doctors, nurses, and other health personnel go all over the world, treating the sick and teaching in their specialties. Engineers, architects, and others build roads, dams, bridges, hospitals, and schools abroad.

Education is free. The percentage of people who graduate from high schools, colleges, and universities in Cuba is higher than in the United States. Since more of the population of Cuba is dark skinned than in the US, their successes contrast sharply with our educational statistics when race is factored in. Cuban teachers are working to abolish illiteracy and expand public education in Africa, South America, and Central America.

During the so-called "special period," when the Soviet Union collapsed and the US forced the former USSR countries to boycott Cuba, Cuba lost 75% of its markets overnight. At the same time, the US tightened its blockade in an attempt to starve the people. The

Cuban government distributed food and other essentials equally to everyone. No one starved, but people tell me they were hungry. There is enough food now and no one goes hungry, because food and other essentials are still distributed to those in need, and organic fruits and vegetables cost almost nothing.

Art, music, and drama, as well as baseball and other sports events are available to all at very low cost.

It was recently reported by an international agency that drug use and addiction in Cuba is the lowest in the hemisphere. Bush immediately said he didn't believe the statistics.

My friends in Cuba would like more money and more things, of course. Remember Rivas, the Cuban psychiatrist who attended the ITAA conference in Oaxaca? His car is 25 cars old and Russian. It breaks down constantly. He'd love a newer, non-Russian car, but he'll never be able to afford one. Cubans need extra bedrooms and new tile for their bathrooms. Buses are terrible. I think that all families have telephones and TVs, given to them by the government, but everyone would like to own a personal computer and a digital camera. I met a young man who was earning money by climbing palm trees, posing for tourists, and selling coconuts. He told me he would give anything to go to Florida, where he would be rich. I asked what he thought he would do to become rich and he didn't know.

I am sure there are professional people and others with good job skills who would like a chance at selfishness, a chance to earn lots of money and spend it on themselves. But no one I know wants Cuba to return to capitalism. They do not want to end their government's altruism. They are proud of what Cubans are accomplishing for the world.

The Cubans I know love Fidel Castro and hope for his recovery. Hugo Chavez of Venezuela visits regularly and always announces, "I am no doctor, but Fidel looks much healthier today." The people smile as they quote him. When a Spanish oncologist told the press that Castro had no sign of cancer, the people were jubilant. I heard them talking excitedly about this in the hospital, in the streets, and in front of my apartment house, where they gather in the evening to gossip. In June 2007 I received excited, happy e-mails after Castro gave his first TV speech since his illness.

My friends believe that Cuba is currently in good hands. They like Raul Castro and the ministers who rule with him. They would like an end to the blockade. Good trade relations would be advantageous to both countries.

How Do We Change Ourselves?

Selfishness.

Like others in the world, you may want to earn as much money as you can and spend it all on yourself and your children. You may love what capitalism has done for you. If it weren't for capitalism, I would not have been able to go to Cuba to give free workshops. And yet I know that my selfishness and my compliance help destroy the world. Until people evolve past selfishness, enforced altruism is the only way I know to save the people on this planet.

Evil.

We must first acknowledge the existence of evil in ourselves. Bill Cornell wrote in the January Transactional Analysis Journal, "If we do not learn to face our hatreds, there will be no true hope or trust." Our individual hates may be based on past hates, may be inherited from our families, or be a response to fear. It may be the way we get excitement or a sense of power, closeness, and camaraderie with other haters.

When we acknowledge the Evil Child, the next step may be no more than deciding on an Adult level, "No matter how much I hate, I will not knowingly harm another human being." Hopefully we will go beyond this and be repulsed by our own Evil Child. We will forgive ourselves for past hates and change hate to compassion. This can be done with or without therapy.

I have an example of a private redecision. Juan told me, "When I was a much younger man, I was a member of a medical team in Africa. Some locals asked me if I'd like to go big game hunting with them and I agreed enthusiastically. I borrowed an army rifle with a first class sight and we were off. In the jungle I was enjoying aiming and looking far into the distance for big game, when suddenly I saw a monkey just a few meters from me, right in my sight. He didn't try to escape. He put his hands over his eyes and cried out, the saddest cry I have ever heard. I dropped the rifle and knew I would never aim a rifle again. I'll never kill an animal or a person." I asked him what he would do if Americans invaded Cuba. He shook his head wearily. "So many will die." He says he would not try to kill anyone.

I am going to suggest an experiment for all of us. We are here in this room. Outside the room are people who may break in to torture and kill all of us or some of us. That is not totally farfetched. Fundamentalist missionaries in Central America are telling their converts that psychologists, like brujos and curanderos (witch doctors and medicine men), are Satanists. Imagine that they have taken over the world and are here to do some mopping up. Or imagine that outside the door is the Argentinean military from the years when they were "disappearing" their intellectuals. Did you know that during that era psychologists were on their hit list and were "disappeared?" People like you and me were tortured to death just because they were psychotherapists.

Here we are in this room, an island. The enemy is outside. Shut your eyes and imagine that they may invade us, even though we are peaceful people. They have unlimited arms and we don't. Imagine that they are an imperial army, the most lethal army in the world. Their leader has convinced them that we are terrorists or dangerous because we are communists. We may be murdered. We may be taken to prisons away from our families, where we will be tortured for months or years.

Millions of people in the world live with this fear, and other millions live where torture, military kidnappings, and killings are daily occurrences.

Prejudice.

I love my friends in Cuba just as I love you, my friends in ITAA. I know that some of you may be prejudiced against atheists, poor people, Castro, or communism. I hope you will give up these prejudices. One way to offset the prejudiced Parent is to make friends with the people you are supposed to hate. Remember the song from South Pacific:

"You've got to be taught to hate and fear
You've got to be taught from year to year

(Here I change it slightly)
To hate all the people your government hates
You've got to be carefully taught."

I want to introduce you to some of my Cuban friends with the hope that you will understand why I care so much for their safety. I wish you could meet Rivas' grandson. He's eleven, handsome and also cute in his white karate outfit. Sometimes he watches baseball games or soap opera in my apartment, while Rivas and I chat. It is unthinkable that American soldiers may someday break into his home and murder this child.

Celeste is loud and funny, bitterly anti-American as always. She is the woman I wrote about in *Explore the World Alone,* who was married to the famous modern artist, Mariano, and worked for the revolution from the time she was eighteen years old. She's now older and more fragile, has trouble walking, but still sings "Gracias a la vida que me ha dado tanto" (thanks to life that has given me so much.) There's a senior center with free lunches near her home, and she and her friends gather there at noon to eat lunch and have discussions. They are studying the World's Great Books, translated into Spanish in large print and sometimes abridged so that a book can be read in two weeks. Because of the paper shortage, books are loaned by the government and then redistributed to another center. Twice a month the seniors have an outing to a beach, museum, or nearby interesting town. They are taken without charge to matinee performances of ballet, symphony, opera, and theater, and to programs given by youth groups, who are very talented.

If the United States invades, Celeste says she will be in the front lines with a gun or rocks. "I'll die fighting for Cuba." (Actually, I cannot imagine how she would get to the front lines in her condition, but I can imagine her, rocks or gun in hand, on her front steps facing the invaders and yelling at them in her old, loud communist voice.)

There is Carlos, a psychiatrist who calls himself my chronic patient because he likes to learn my work by experiencing it. In March, during my final Cuban workshop, I had him put his stomach in a chair, be the stomach, and let his stomach talk. He was delighted, and said that it is a technique he can use with his psychosomatic patients. There is the psychologist Greta, small and square, with a great laugh. In her spare time, of which she has very little, she arranges comedies and musical evenings for hospital staff and patients. And Tony, my translator, who sometimes has to ask for a break after translating a piece of work, because he is so affected by it. And Adrienne, a Canadian who went to Cuba after the revolution, married the American who was head of the US news service, and stayed.

There's Juan and Juan's gorgeous Black granddaughter, sixteen, a student in a special pre-medical secondary school. A bus picks her up every Sunday night and brings her home on Fridays. Books, uniforms, room and board, everything is free. What would happen to her dreams if we should conquer Cuba? Before the Revolution, many black children received only three years of public schooling in shacks where they wrote their lessons with sticks in the dirt. Do you think the Florida Cubans, who took their money and left, rather than remain in an altruistic society, would give a damn about a young Black adolescent who wants to be a doctor?

These are only a few of the people I know and love. I don't want anything to happen to them! I hope you will insist that we begin trade relationships with Cuba, not war.

I haven't mentioned Iraq. I know that if I had taught there, I would have Iraqi friends as dear to me as my Cuban friends and my ITAA friends. What more can I say? I am hurting both for our country and for the world.

I close with two quotes. The first is about another of our wars of aggression, which most people have forgotten, our war against the Philippines. In three years we killed thousands and thousands of people. I suppose we believed we were there to give them democracy or freedom or something else that they did not want from us. President McKinley, like our current president, assured Americans that God had spoken to him and said He was on our side. The arrogance!

On A Soldier Fallen In the Philippines
by William Vaughn Moody

"Let him never dream that his bullet's scream
Went wide of its island mark,

Home to the heart of his darling land,
Where she stumbled and sinned in the dark."

The second quote is from the Himeyuri Peace Museum, Okinawa. Bob Goulding and I did a workshop in Okinawa in the mid 1970s and helped the people say belated goodbyes to their dead from World War II. Five years ago I returned for a final workshop there and some of the original participants, all now retired, attended for old time's sake. One of them had said goodbye to her father at the first workshop. This time she said goodbye to a sister who died a few months before the workshop. She is a Christian, so sang *Amazing Grace* in Japanese after her goodbye.

Here is the quote:

"A war does not simply erupt out of nothing. It is a tragedy of our own making, and we should be able to prevent it. Why do we have to kill each other on this small planet called earth, a small fragile ecosystem in which plants, animals, and human beings have no choice but to coexist peacefully or perish together?"

We must focus on eliminating our own prejudice, replacing evil with compassion, selfishness with altruism, and compliance with courage. When we do this, we can help our clients do the same.

References:

1. Eric Berne, MD, *What Do You Say After You Say Hello?*, Grove Press, New York, 1972.
2. William F. Cornell, "The Inevitability of Uncertainty," *Transactional Analysis Journal*, Vol. 37 No.1, 2007.
3. Bob Dylan, "George Jackson," a song, 1971.
4. Himeyuri Peace Museum, Okinawa, Japan, 1950.
5. William Vaughn Moody, "On A Soldier Fallen in the Philippines", *Modern American Poetry*, Harcourt Brace and Howe, 1919.
6. Miguel de Unamuno, speech, University of Salamanca, 1936.
7. Philip Zimbardo, *The Lucifer Effect*, Random House, NY, 2007.

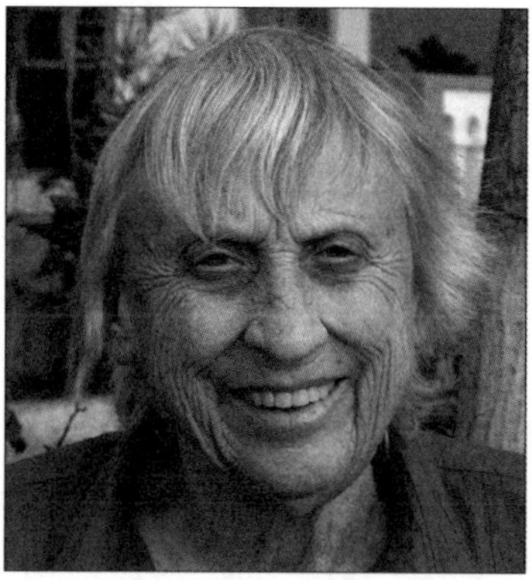

Photo by Inger Acking

Mary Goulding, MSW, is a Teaching Member of the International Transactional Analysis Association and a founder of the Redecision Therapy Association. She and her husband, the late Robert L. Goulding, MD, developed Redecision therapy, a system of brief psychotherapy based on transactional analysis theory and their own redecision techniques. For over twenty years they co-directed the Western Institute For Group and Family Therapy in Watsonville, California, and taught psychotherapists across the world.

Mary Goulding is one of three women and the only social worker to be honored by the Milton Erickson Foundation as a major presenter at all of the Evolution of Psychotherapy conferences. She has lectured and presented workshops at ITAA, AGPA, and both APAs, as well as at colleges and universities. She is the author of eight books.